ENDOCRINOLOGY RESEARCH AND CLINICAL DEVELOPMENTS

POLYCYSTIC OVARY SYNDROME

CAUSES, DIAGNOSIS AND MANAGEMENT

ENDOCRINOLOGY RESEARCH AND CLINICAL DEVELOPMENTS

Additional books and e-books in this series can be found on Nova's website under the Series tab.

Endocrinology Research and Clinical Developments

Polycystic Ovary Syndrome

Causes, Diagnosis and Management

Katherine Webb
Editor

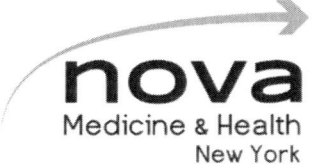

Copyright © 2021 by Nova Science Publishers, Inc.

All rights reserved. No part of this book may be reproduced, stored in a retrieval system or transmitted in any form or by any means: electronic, electrostatic, magnetic, tape, mechanical photocopying, recording or otherwise without the written permission of the Publisher.

We have partnered with Copyright Clearance Center to make it easy for you to obtain permissions to reuse content from this publication. Simply navigate to this publication's page on Nova's website and locate the "Get Permission" button below the title description. This button is linked directly to the title's permission page on copyright.com. Alternatively, you can visit copyright.com and search by title, ISBN, or ISSN.

For further questions about using the service on copyright.com, please contact:
Copyright Clearance Center
Phone: +1-(978) 750-8400   Fax: +1-(978) 750-4470   E-mail: info@copyright.com

NOTICE TO THE READER

The Publisher has taken reasonable care in the preparation of this book, but makes no expressed or implied warranty of any kind and assumes no responsibility for any errors or omissions. No liability is assumed for incidental or consequential damages in connection with or arising out of information contained in this book. The Publisher shall not be liable for any special, consequential, or exemplary damages resulting, in whole or in part, from the readers' use of, or reliance upon, this material. Any parts of this book based on government reports are so indicated and copyright is claimed for those parts to the extent applicable to compilations of such works.

Independent verification should be sought for any data, advice or recommendations contained in this book. In addition, no responsibility is assumed by the Publisher for any injury and/or damage to persons or property arising from any methods, products, instructions, ideas or otherwise contained in this publication.

This publication is designed to provide accurate and authoritative information with regard to the subject matter covered herein. It is sold with the clear understanding that the Publisher is not engaged in rendering legal or any other professional services. If legal or any other expert assistance is required, the services of a competent person should be sought. FROM A DECLARATION OF PARTICIPANTS JOINTLY ADOPTED BY A COMMITTEE OF THE AMERICAN BAR ASSOCIATION AND A COMMITTEE OF PUBLISHERS.

Additional color graphics may be available in the e-book version of this book.

Library of Congress Cataloging-in-Publication Data

ISBN: 978-1-53619-527-9

Published by Nova Science Publishers, Inc. † New York

CONTENTS

Preface vii

Chapter 1 An Update on Low-Grade Inflammation and
Oxidative Stress, as Consequences of Insulin
Resistance and Hyperandrogenism, in the
Pathogenesis of Polycystic Ovary Syndrome 1
*Poopak Eftekhari-Yazdi, Nahid Nasiri,
Fatemeh Hassani and Arezoo Arabipoor*

Chapter 2 An Overview of Possible Health Risk and
Complications of Polycystic Ovary Syndrome 77
*Iram Ashaq Kawa, Akbar Masood,
Shahnaz Ahmad Mir, Saika Manzoor
and Fouzia Rashid*

Chapter 3 Polycystic Ovary Syndrome:
A Fresh Insight in Relation to Its Inflammatory
and Coagulatory Pathophysiology 127
*Saika Manzoor, Khalid Bashir Dar,
Mohd Ashraf Ganie, Iram Ashaq Kawa
and Fouzia Rashid*

Index 169

PREFACE

This work contains three chapters, each examining the hormonal imbalance disease polycystic ovary syndrome (PCOS) from a different perspective. Chapter 1 describes various characteristics of PCOS and reviews recent approaches for treatment strategies, including antioxidant supplementation, anti-inflammatory agents, and lifestyle modification. Chapter 2 reviews possible health risks and complications of PCOS. Finally, Chapter 3 aims to provide an understanding and wider concept of pathogenesis and intricacy of various pathways pertaining to the heterogeneity of this syndrome that can help to comprehend the disease's progression in detail.

Chapter 1 - Polycystic ovary syndrome (PCOS), as the most frequent hormonal imbalance disease and endocrinopathy causing infertility, is characterized by insulin resistance, glucose intolerance, hyperandrogenism, obesity, cardiovascular problems, and obesity-independent dyslipidemia. As a systemic, polygenic, polyfactorial, and autoimmune disease, PCOS involves a chronic low-grade inflammation which plays a key role in ovulatory dysfunction, and the pathogenesis of the disease. The ovarian overproduction of androgens, as the main characteristics of PCOS, is responsible for causing severe symptoms such as insulin resistance, hirsutism, and infertility. Hyperandrogenism may activate the blood immune mononuclear cells (MNC), as proinflammatory cytokines-secreting cells, increases their sensitivity to glucose and promote diet-dependent low-grade inflammation in PCOS. Therefore, a battery of high-carbohydrate intake, insulin resistance, and hyperandrogenism can be considered initiators of inflammation in this disease. Noteworthy, it was also reported that increased levels of reactive oxygen species (ROS) in granulosa cells (GCs) and follicular fluid may affect oocyte quality and pregnancy results in PCOS patients who underwent ART (assisted reproductive technology) cycles. Therefore, effects of antioxidants and anti-inflammatory agents in the treatment of PCOS patients have been examined; however, the results of such studies are still under debate. In the present chapter, the authors look at the presence of inflammatory mediators including glucose-stimulated tumor necrosis factor-α (TNFα, a known mediator of insulin resistance), interleukin (IL)-1β, IL-6, IL-18, E-selectin, ICAM-1 and VCAM-1, C-reactive protein (CRP), and activated nuclear factor-κB (NFκB) and its inhibitor, IκBα protein (which were all shown by animal and human studies to be involved in PCOS etiology), in patients' blood serum and follicular fluid follow a diet high in saturated fat. Then, the authors discuss the pathophysiological roles of chronic low-grade inflammation in the presence and absence of obesity. The authors also present how inflammation may affect the dynamic of folliculogenesis - follicle maturation and arrest- and thereby, the pathophysiology of the ovary. Finally, recent approaches including antioxidant supplementation, anti-inflammatory agents, and lifestyle modification as potentially more effective treatment strategies for PCOS women who underwent ART cycles, are reviewed.

Chapter 2 - Polycystic Ovary Syndrome (PCOS) is the most common disorder associated with a spectrum of endocrine, reproductive, metabolic and psychological features. It affects millions of women worldwide and represents a major burden on health and economy. PCOS women are usually diagnosed in adolescence or in early adulthood with signs of hirsutism, acne or oligomenorrhea or when presenting for treatment of infertility. However, the health issues associated with PCOS go well beyond the management of these typical symptoms and likely persist throughout the reproductive years and beyond menopause which significantly affects the quality of life of these women. Amidst its prevalence and repercussions for metabolic, reproductive and psychological wellbeing PCOS remains under-diagnosed; partly because of the heterogeneity of the phenotypes presented by the syndrome. The phenotypes vary significantly depending on the stage of life, ethnicity, genotype and environmental factors like Body Mass Index and lifestyle. Although the pathogenesis of this syndrome remains elusive, abnormalities in action or secretion of gonadotropin, steroidogenesis, folliculogenesis, insulin action or secretion among others contribute to its development. The dysregulation of these diverse systems is thought to result from genetic, epigenetic and environmental factors. A better understanding of these factors is important for the determination of preventive risk factors and effective treatment of this syndrome. The primary concern of this complex disorder is timely diagnosis; education of patients and healthcare professionals; screening and treatment for complications that would reduce the health and economic burden associated with PCOS and its related co-morbid conditions. Keeping in view the complexity of this syndrome and the impact on the quality of life of these women, this chapter will try to shed some light on the clinical presentation, diagnosis and pathogenesis of PCOS. This chapter will also present a general overview on complications and associated health risks of this syndrome.

Chapter 3 - PCOS is a multi-factorial complex disorder affecting various organ systems of the body. It is a vicious cycle, when it gets triggered at any unknown point; it results in full-blown metabolic syndrome. The diverse etiology of PCOS adversely affects various pathways like insulin resistance, lipid metabolism, steroidogenesis, inflammation, and coagulation cascade. Long-term risk factors associated with this disorder are T2DM, glucose intolerance, CVD, VTE, pulmonary embolism, infertility, pregnancy complications, cancer, etc. PCOS shoots beyond the scope of endocrine and reproductive abnormalities and is considered as a syndrome associated with metabolic dysfunctioning of the body. It can be considered, as an umbrella with a gallop of troubles underneath it. Therefore, its management requires collaborative efforts like lifestyle intervention i.e., eating habits, physical activities, use of medications, counseling, aesthetic approach and psychotherapies, etc. PCOS requires proper evaluation procedures to rule out its symptoms overlapping with other disease conditions. Various clinical symptoms that appear with the onset of disease are an indication of the underlying pathologies associated with PCOS. The main aim of this chapter is to provide an understanding and wider concept of pathogenesis and intricacy of various pathways pertaining to the heterogeneity of this syndrome that can help to comprehend the disease's progression in detail, especially in relation to the involvement of various inflammatory pathways and coagulatory disturbances which build up over time and can have serious implications for the overall health of the concerned individual. There is a crucial role of mechanisms like abnormal hypothalamus-pituitary-ovarian axis, hormonal imbalance, insulin resistance, hyperinsulinemia, deregulated production of inflammatory cytokines, and coagulatory factors in PCOS pathogenesis. Targeting these cascades for devising effective therapeutic management against such a far-reaching disorder could prove a beneficent strategy. Comprehensive knowledge added in this chapter will provide sufficient information pertaining to varied aspects of this disorder like various symptoms, different criteria, prevalence, reproductive, endocrine, cardiac, hematological, inflammatory, and coagulatory features, long-term outcomes, and the possible root causes of pathogenesis in this syndrome.

In: Polycystic Ovary Syndrome
Editor: Katherine Webb

ISBN: 978-1-53619-527-9
© 2021 Nova Science Publishers, Inc.

Chapter 1

AN UPDATE ON LOW-GRADE INFLAMMATION AND OXIDATIVE STRESS, AS CONSEQUENCES OF INSULIN RESISTANCE AND HYPERANDROGENISM, IN THE PATHOGENESIS OF POLYCYSTIC OVARY SYNDROME

Poopak Eftekhari-Yazdi[1,*], PhD, Nahid Nasiri[1], PhD, Fatemeh Hassani[1], PhD and Arezoo Arabipoor[2]

[1]Department of Embryology, Reproductive Biomedicine Research Center, Royan Institute for Reproductive Biomedicine, ACECR, Tehran, Iran

[2]Department of Endocrinology and Female Infertility, Reproductive Biomedicine Research Center, Royan Institute for Reproductive Biomedicine, ACECR, Tehran, Iran

---

* Corresponding Author's E-mail: eftekhari@royaninstitute.org.

ABSTRACT

Polycystic ovary syndrome (PCOS), as the most frequent hormonal imbalance disease and endocrinopathy causing infertility, is characterized by insulin resistance, glucose intolerance, hyperandrogenism, obesity, cardiovascular problems, and obesity-independent dyslipidemia. As a systemic, polygenic, polyfactorial, and autoimmune disease, PCOS involves a chronic low-grade inflammation which plays a key role in ovulatory dysfunction, and the pathogenesis of the disease. The ovarian overproduction of androgens, as the main characteristics of PCOS, is responsible for causing severe symptoms such as insulin resistance, hirsutism, and infertility. Hyperandrogenism may activate the blood immune mononuclear cells (MNC), as proinflammatory cytokines-secreting cells, increases their sensitivity to glucose and promote diet-dependent low-grade inflammation in PCOS. Therefore, a battery of high-carbohydrate intake, insulin resistance, and hyperandrogenism can be considered initiators of inflammation in this disease.

Noteworthy, it was also reported that increased levels of reactive oxygen species (ROS) in granulosa cells (GCs) and follicular fluid may affect oocyte quality and pregnancy results in PCOS patients who underwent ART (assisted reproductive technology) cycles. Therefore, effects of antioxidants and anti-inflammatory agents in the treatment of PCOS patients have been examined; however, the results of such studies are still under debate.

In the present chapter, we look at the presence of inflammatory mediators including glucose-stimulated tumor necrosis factor-α (TNFα, a known mediator of insulin resistance), interleukin (IL)-1β, IL-6, IL-18, E-selectin, ICAM-1 and VCAM-1, C-reactive protein (CRP), and activated nuclear factor-κB (NFκB) and its inhibitor, IκBα protein (which were all shown by animal and human studies to be involved in PCOS etiology), in patients' blood serum and follicular fluid follow a diet high in saturated fat. Then, we discuss the pathophysiological roles of chronic low-grade inflammation in the presence and absence of obesity. We also present how inflammation may affect the dynamic of folliculogenesis - follicle maturation and arrest- and thereby, the pathophysiology of the ovary. Finally, recent approaches including antioxidant supplementation, anti-inflammatory agents, and lifestyle modification as potentially more effective treatment strategies for PCOS women who underwent ART cycles, are reviewed.

INTRODUCTION

Polycystic ovary syndrome (PCOS) is the most frequent hormonal imbalance disease and endocrinopathy that causes infertility with high heterogeneity, and affects up to 10% of premenopausal women. Clinical features of PCOS include insulin resistance (IR), glucose intolerance, hyperandrogenism (HA), secondary amenorrhea, obesity (particularly visceral adiposity), cardiovascular problems, and obesity-independent dyslipidemia. These clinical features all change with age [1, 2]. The modified Rotterdom criteria characterizes PCOS as the observation of two out of the subsequent three criteria: polycystic appearance of ovaries by ultrasound; clinical or biochemical HA; and anovulation or oligoovulation [3]. PCOS is an important long-term public health disease accompanied by psychological, metabolic, and reproductive dysfunction, which causes this disease to affect the adulthood lifestyle and is accompanied by infertility in 70% to 80% of patients [4]. A hyperandrogenic environment alongside a low grade inflammatory status in PCOS ovaries may induce altered folliculogenesis, and contribute to infertility from anovulation [5, 6].

Therapeutic protocols for PCOS management are based on its clinical symptoms and mainly include attenuation of IR, ovulation induction, and androgen adjustment [7].

1. LOW GRADE INFLAMMATION AND AN ALTERED REACTIVE OXYGEN SPECIES (ROS) STATE IN POLYCYSTIC OVARY SYNDROME (PCOS)

In 2001, Kelly et al. introduced low-grade chronic inflammation as a new mechanism in the development and immunopathogenesis of PCOS [8]. It is a systemic, polygenic, polyfactorial, autoimmune disease with associated complications that include ovulatory dysfunction, coronary heart disease, IR, and type 2 diabetes [9].

The presence of classic inflammatory markers such as C-reactive protein (CRP), interleukin-6 (IL-6), IL-18, tumor necrosis factor (TNF), acute phase serum amyloid A (APSAA) and monocyte chemotactic protein-1 (MCP-1) provide clues for an association between PCOS and inflammation [10, 11].

1.1. C-Reactive Protein (CRP)

Among the suggested inflammatory mediators, CRP is a biomarker that participates in a broad-spectrum of inflammatory responses and has many clinical applications [12]. The results of recent studies showed elevated CRP levels in PCOS patients [12, 13]. Data from a meta-analysis of 31 articles that compared PCOS (n=2359) versus healthy women (n=1289) showed that CRP, among other inflammatory mediators, was 96% higher in PCOS patients compared to the control women. The results reported by this meta-analysis indicated a relation between CRP and body mass index (BMI) where an increased CRP concentration might be linked to overweight in these patients [14].

1.2. Interleukin-6 (IL-6)

IL-6 is another cytokine secreted by adipose tissue that plays a role in the development of inflammation in PCOS [15] There is a link between increased concentrations of IL-6 and total testosterone, obesity, and IR in PCOS patients. Therefore, IL-6 can be an appropriate biomarker for the diagnosis of PCOS [16, 17].

A meta-analysis of 20 articles (n=1618 women) was conducted to evaluate IL-6 levels in patients with PCOS. According to the results, PCOS patients had increased levels of IL-6 compared to healthy subjects who were matched for BMI. A link existed between elevated IL-6 concentrations and total testosterone, as well IR in women with PCOS compared to healthy women. Based on the findings of the meta-analysis, elevated levels of IL-6 were not considered to be among the main features of PCOS in women;

however, in terms of therapeutic measures, IL-6 could be considered as an appropriate biomarker [16].

1.3. Tumor Necrosis Factor Alpha (TNF-α)

The importance of TNF-α in the pathogenesis of IR, diabetes, and obesity has been reported [18]. TNF-α mediated downregulation of glucose transporter type 4 (GLUT4) may be responsible for impaired glucose transport into cells, which can occur in conditions such as IR [19]. Elevated TNF-α levels are associated with an increase in the number of ovarian follicles and follicular hyperplasia, reduced ovulation rate, and decreased progesterone production in PCOS patients who underwent in vitro fertilization (IVF) [20, 21].

1.4. Interleukin-18 (IL-18)

The close relation between IL-18 and PCOS was evaluated in several studies. In 2011, Yang et al. reported that PCOS women had significant elevations in serum IL-18 levels compared with healthy individuals [22]. Günther et al., in 2016, stated that elevations in weight could be accompanied by increased serum and follicular fluid levels of IL-18 [23]. According to their results, a link exists between the ovarian stimulation response and follicular fluid content of IL-18 in ART ovarian stimulation protocols, which plays a key role in subsequent pregnancy success [23].

1.5. Cell Adhesion Molecules (CAMs)

The role of cell adhesion molecules (CAMs) such as E-selectin, endothelin 1, intercellular cell adhesion molecule-1 (ICAM1), and vascular cell adhesion molecule-1 (VCAM1) in induction of chronic low-grade inflammation and endothelial dysfunction is well-known [24]. Both diabetics and PCOS patients have increased levels of systemic adhesion molecules [25]. ICAM-1 and VCAM-1 expressions have been specifically investigated in the granulosa and theca cell layer in PCOS-like mouse models; the results showed increased expressions of these CAMs [26, 27]. Based on the results obtained from recent studies, local silencing of VCAM-1 and other molecules involved in cell adhesion and the inflammatory process might be potential treatment strategies and provide promise for future management of PCOS [26].

Recently, reduced levels of osteoprotegerin, a non-classic marker of inflammation that inhibits apoptosis and decreases inflammation [28, 29]; increased levels of mean platelet volume (MPV), an indicator of platelet aggregation [30]; and high amounts of advanced glycation end products (AGEs), as an inflammatory mediator in IR, obesity and PCOS [31] have been reported. Ferritin is another low-grade inflammatory marker. Elevations in ferritin have been reported for PCOS patients who have IR and/or obesity [32]. However, increased circulating levels of some inflammatory mediators, such as CRP, in lean PCOS women, indicates that the inflammation is independent from obesity in these patients [33-35].

Oxidative stress (OS) is an imbalance between the oxidant, as free radicals or reactive oxygen species (ROS) derived from the aerobic metabolism, and antioxidants that protect the body from the harmful effects of ROS. OS induces changes that include DNA damage, apoptosis, necrosis, and cell death, in addition to epigenetic alterations carried out by DNA methylation [36, 37].

ROS hypoxia-inducible factor-1 (HIF-1) and activated protein-1 (AP-1) can trigger the release of pro-inflammatory cytokines and induce an inflammatory response by activating the signaling pathways of nuclear factor-κB (NF-κB), as a master regulator of inflammation in mammalian cells [38]. The close connection between OS and inflammation makes it difficult to distinguish between them [39].

A relationship exists between OS and cancer and chronic disorders such as cardiovascular disease, diabetes and PCOS [40]. According to the eevidence, OS and PCOS play roles in different aspects of natural female reproduction and the outcomes of assisted reproduction techniques (ARTs) [41].

Different signaling pathways in inflammatory diseases are affected by OS; thereby, it is difficult to ascertain the same OS markers for these diseases. The results of recent studies show that PCOS patients, because of their determined mitochondrial dysfunction and decreased antioxidant protection [42, 43], have elevated levels of the OS markers malondialdehyde (MDA), glutathione peroxidase (GPx), superoxide dismutase (SOD), asymmetric dimethyl arginine (AMDA), and paraoxonase-1 (PON1) [44-46]. For this reason, PCOS patients are at increased risk for breast, endometrial, and ovarian cancers [47].

It remains to be determined if the altered OS levels in patients arise from PCOS or from PCOS complications. However, we have reported that abdominal obesity can induce both systemic and follicular fluid OS that is independent from PCOS [43]. Obesity and metabolic disorders in PCOS women may be the most significant factors for reduction of total antioxidant capacity (TAC) levels, mitochondrial dysfunction, OS, and inflammation [48]. However, conflicting reports indicate that non-obese infertile PCOS patients have higher levels of MDA and systemic OS during the ICSI process compared to non-obese infertile patients without PCOS [49].

Next, we intend to discuss the role of different PCOS complications in OS induction. Because PCOS is always accompanied by one or more of these complications, OS seems to be an inseparable part of this disease.

2. ASSOCIATION OF OBESITY AND DYSLIPIDEMIA WITH THE OXIDATIVE STRESS (OS)/ INFLAMMATORY STATE IN POLYCYSTIC OVARY SYNDROME (PCOS)

Obesity is a common phenotype in PCOS patients and it accounts for 42% of those who are obese [50].

Based on the available literature, abdominal obesity or visceral accumulation of adipose tissue plays a more significant role in the etiology of metabolic syndromes and is highly correlated with PCOS rather than general obesity (subcutaneous adiposity) [50, 51]. Abdominal obesity is estimated in 40%-80% of women with PCOS and in 50% of PCOS patients with normal BMI [52]. In addition, there is a well-defined link between OS and obesity (both general and abdominal) [53, 54]. Increased adipokine levels and decreased adiponectin levels, as markers of low-grade inflammation, are correlated with dyslipidemia in PCOS [55]. Mild hypercholesterolemia and other lipid patterns are present in PCOS women. Approximately 70% of PCOS patients show various levels of dyslipidemia. Hypercholesterolemia is identified by elevations in triglycerides (TG), lipoprotein concentrations and total cholesterol (TC), in addition to low levels of high-density lipoprotein cholesterol (HDL-C) and low-density lipoprotein cholesterol (LDL-C), and has been defined for PCOS associated dyslipidemia [56, 57]. Hypercholesterolemia is concomitant with OS [58, 59]. Therefore, lipid and protein peroxidation markers in obese PCOS women that are significantly altered and correlate with mild hypercholesterolemia include increased oxidized low-density lipoprotein (ox-LDL), advanced oxidation protein products (AOPP), thiobarbituric reactive substances (TBARS), and MDA, as well as decreased copper-zinc-containing SOD (CuZn-SOD) and glutathione peroxidase (GSHPx) [60-62].

In a regulatory feedback cycle, PCOS-involved dyslipidemia can exacerbate other PCOS complications, which include HA, OS, and IR, and promote the pathophysiology of PCOS and propagate infertility in these patients. The results from different studies of ART indicate that obesity can alter both oocyte quality and pre-implantation embryo development, and this change mainly occurs via mitochondrial dysfunction, apoptosis and lipotoxicity-induced endoplasmic reticulum stress [63].

3. INSULIN RESISTANCE (IR) ACCOMPANIES THE INFLAMMATORY/OXIDATIVE STRESS (OS) STATE IN POLYCYSTIC OVARY SYNDROME (PCOS)

PCOS is a chronic systemic disease and its pathogenesis mechanism is highly accompanied by OS, IR, and HA [64-66]. The results of numerous studies have shown a frequent association between chronic inflammation and OS with obesity, IR and HA in PCOS patients [43, 67, 68]. The association between IR and obesity is one of the most prominent. Up to 50% of obese patients have IR; thereby, IR is one of the major mechanisms by which excess adiposity contributes to OS [50]. In addition, these two pathologic phenotypes, IR and obesity, are strongly concomitant with dyslipidemia [69, 70]. Numerous reports show the same lipid profile of increased triglycerides and decreased HDL-C for PCOS associated dyslipidemia and PCOS associated IR [71]; despite the frequent co-occurrence of obesity and IR, their role in PCOS pathogenesis is independent of each other [1, 2].

IR is a physiological disorder during which the biological effect of a defined concentration of insulin is less than expected and it affects 50%-70% of PCOS patients [71, 72]. In the presence of IR, the cells fail to properly respond to insulin, which leads to disruptions in glucose metabolism that include compensatory hyperglycemia and hyperinsulinemia [72]. IR-induced hyperglycemia leads to increased ROS production; hence, PCOS-associated IR is usually correlated with observation of OS markers such as decreased glutathione (GSH) and increased MDA, nonesterified fatty acid (NEFA), and protein carbonyl [73-75]. Reciprocally, OS plays a critical role in IR pathogenesis and OS has an inhibitory effect on insulin signaling [76]. Moreover, the protective effect of antioxidants such as N-acetylcysteine (NAC), vitamin E, and α-lipoic acid on insulin sensitivity implies that these antioxidant compounds could be used in therapeutic protocols [77, 78].

Inflammation and OS in PCOS-associated IR are mainly formed through post-insulin receptor defects. While insulin receptors in PCOS are usually normal, insulin receptor substrate (IRS) plays a key role in IR pathogenesis [79, 80]. In OS, the IRS is abnormally phosphorylated and inhibited by certain activated protein kinases which reduce its capacity for normal binding to the insulin receptor. This phenomenon prevents the activation of downstream effectors such as phosphatidyl inositol 3-kinase (PI3K) and disrupts normal insulin signaling [81]. Disruptions in insulin signaling subsequently promote IR, which then causes compensatory hyperinsulinemia. Subsequently, hyperinsulinemia can propagate luteinizing hormone- (LH) stimulated androgen production both via androgen receptors and/or insulin growth factor (IGF-1) receptors, induce ovarian HA in PCOS patients, and cause abnormal ovary function [82, 83]. Thus, HA can originate from IR in PCOS [84].

4. THE RELATIONSHIP BETWEEN INSULIN RESISTANCE (IR), HYPERANDROGENISM (HA) AND INFLAMMATION IN POLYCYSTIC OVARY SYNDROME (PCOS)

HA is a common classical feature of PCOS that is diagnosed in 70%-80% of patients [85]. Despite the lack of clarity about the role of HA in PCOS pathogenesis, the presence of HA along with inflammation, OS markers, obesity and IR are well-defined [86, 87]. Therefore, it has been reported that TNF-α, a known inflammatory marker can mainly trigger androgen production in rat ovaries [88] by NF-κB signaling [89, 90]. The inappropriate reaction of abnormal ovarian theca cells to ROS may promote the HA state in ovaries [91], which has been verified by the presence of increased adiposity, and enhanced levels of TG, NEFA, fasting blood glucose (FBG), fasting serum insulin (FINS), and homeostasis model assessment of insulin resistance (HOMA-IR), and altered OS markers such as SOD, MDA and GSH in animal models of androgen-induced PCOS. This finding showed the close link between HA, inflammation, and obesity in PCOS [92-94]. The logical explanation for the pathologic sequence appears to be as follows: OS underlies IR and IR, in turn, causes HA, which may subsequently induce OS and continue this pathogenic feedback cycle that plays a critical role in PCOS pathogenesis. However, OS still accompanies PCOS even in the absence of IR and obesity [95, 96].

5. Disrupted Folliculogenesis in the Inflammatory Environment of Polycystic Ovary Syndrome (PCOS) Ovaries

Women with PCOS frequently exhibit ovarian dysfunction induced subfertility or infertility. Low numbers of mature oocytes and a decreased fertilization and embryo cleavage rates, along with a grade I/II embryo formation rate and high miscarriage rate are the most important reproductive disorders observed in PCOS patients who referred for IVF/ICSI cycles. Ovarian dysfunction associated infertility in these patients is confirmed by a reduction in the mean ovarian total volume and ovary cortex volume due to increased numbers of follicle atresia and reduced numbers of antral follicles, accumulation of small subcortical follicles, elevated mean count of primary and preantral follicles, higher level of estradiol on the hCG administration day and impaired granulosa cell (GC) function [97-99]. GCs participate in different important folliculogenesis events that range from oocyte development and ovulation to fertilization and resultant embryo implantation. GC dysfunction is associated with abnormal folliculogenesis and infertility in PCOS women [100, 101]. In response to the elevated number of small follicles in PCOS ovaries, GCs of the growing follicle begin to secrete increased levels of anti-Müllerian hormone (AMH) [102] that, in the form of negative feedback regulation, reduces FSH levels and finally decreases antral follicle counts as FSH-dependent follicles [103]. However, ovarian disorders in the PCOS may be arise from the presence of any of the factors contributing to the pathogenesis of the disease such as inflammation, IR and HA. For example, significant macrophage and lymphocyte counts in PCOS ovaries are indicative of persistent chronic inflammation that may accompanied by disrupted folliculogenesis [84, 104]. In addition, higher levels of ROS and inflammatory markers such as IL-6 and TNF-α in GCs and follicular fluid of PCOS patients correlate with poor oocyte quality and subsequent subfertility [105].

The thickness of the zona pellucida in the oocytes of PCOS patients is significantly lower than other non-PCOS patients, and it is mainly attributed to a higher rate of apoptosis in GCs, as cells that participate in formation of the zona pellucida. This pathologic event seems to be due to OS [106]. GC apoptosis can cause follicular atresia [107] and is correlated with empty follicle syndrome [108]. On the other hand, intrinsic inflammation and OS in PCOS patients stimulates proliferation of androgen-producing theca cells that leads to increased androgen production by the ovaries [109] and further stimulates the defective cycle in PCOS pathogenesis. Modulating IL-6, MDA and TNF-α via antioxidant and anti-inflammatory compounds can restore ovary volume and function, and the hormonal pattern [5, 110, 111].

Oocyte size and diameter, which may be affected by hyperinsulinemia and HA, is decreased in PCOS patients [112]. In addition, these patients have more insulin receptors compared with healthy women [113, 114], which is due to elevated receptor expression in pre-antral and antral compared with primary and primordial follicles. The observed reduction in oocyte volume may be caused by a hyperinsulinemia state in PCOS patients.

Ovarian hyperinsulinemia also increases testosterone secretion through elevated conversion of progesterone to androstenedione by theca cells, which subsequently converts to testosterone and induces HA [115]. The resultant HA may further increase LH levels, increase ovarian theca cell hyperplasia, and continue the vicious cycle of extra production of androgen and LH. For example, excess androgen stimulates the development of primordial and primary follicles, which express more androgen receptors compared with pre-antral and antral follicles, and then generates increased concentrations of AMH. As noted earlier, this hormonal imbalance may subsequently disturb oocyte development [116] and reduce future chances for fertility.

6. THE OUTCOMES OF ASSISTED REPRODUCTIVE TECHNIQUES IN POLYCYSTIC OVARY SYNDROME (PCOS) PATIENTS: ASSOCIATION BETWEEN INFLAMMATORY/OXIDATIVE STRESS (OS) STATUS AND RESPONSE TO TREATMENT

Despite more retrieved oocytes from PCOS patients during IVF/ICSI cycles, these patients have lower numbers of good quality oocytes, and decreased fertilization, decreased cleavage rate and decreased normal embryo development rates, which alter their clinical outcomes [99].

As previously mentioned, the signs of OS or inflammatory markers in serum and follicular fluid of PCOS patients, as well as oocytes surrounding GCs, have been reported [117-119]. Outcomes of ART treatment include age-realted ovarian dysfunction (ovarian aging), decreased oocyte and embryo quality, and altered fertilization, embryo development and subsequnt pregnancy, which may be influenced by OS factors [117, 120]. As a result, the hypothesis that most cases of ART outcome failure in PCOS patients originates from OS is reinforced.

8-isoprostane (8-IP) is one of the most characterized ART markers that is related to ART outcome in PCOS patients. Its increased level in blood serum is associated with higher abortion rate and pregnancy loss [121]. MDA and total oxidant capacity (TOC) are other provital factors and their serum levels, and, in smaller amounts in follicular fluid of PCOS patients, is closely correlated with embryo quality [122]. During ovarian stimulation, exessive ROS acumulation in GCs may cause GC apoptosis, which is also accompained by empty follicle syndrome, reduced numbers of retrived oocytes and a reduced fertilization rate as well as decreased cleavage and pregnancy rates [123-125].

8-hydroxy-2'-deoxyguanosine (8-OHdG) is a critical OS marker. Reduced levels of 8-OHdG in fluid of dominant follicle in PCOS patients represents their decreased antioxidant defense [121] and is another strong predictor of oocyte maturity and successful fertilization rate in PCOS patients. In comparison with higher ROS production in PCOS tissues, 8-

OHdG levels can accurately predict ART clinical outcomes. However, considering the prominent role of OS and inflammation in PCOS pathogenesis and its ART cycle consequences, it seems that modulation of OS and inflammation should be considered an inseparable part of the future treatment protocols of PCOS-associated infertility.

7. Under Investigation Antioxidants and Anti-Inflammatories Agents in Management of Infertile PCOS Patients

Due to the multifactorial pathogenesis of PCOS, treatment of this endocrinopathy is predominantly symptomatic [126]. The clinical features of PCOs are different and include: reproductive dysfunctions (infertility, pregnancy-related complications), metabolic disorders (obesity, insulin resistance, type II diabetes, hypertension, cardiovascular disease and non-alcoholic fatty liver disease) and psychological features (anxiety, depression, impaired quality of life, body image and eating disorders) [127]. Several infertility management options including life style modification, ovarian induction with letrozole, clomiphene citrate, gonadotropins and in the case of resistance to medicine, laparoscopic ovarian surgery and/or assisted reproductive techniques (ART) were reported. Therefore, the best option for PCOS patients would be a causative treatment; however, due to its heterogeneity, this decision making is difficult task [126]. The aim of current review is to evaluate the recent clinical studies on the actual evidence based therapies including antioxidants, anti-inflammatories, and life style modification to overcome infertility problem and to improve the success rate in PCOS women underwent ART cycles.

7.1. Adjunctive Antioxidants Therapy

The negative impacts of OS and ROS on female reproductive tract have been well investigated over the years [128, 129]. Several proposed mechanisms of actions were reported for supplementary antioxidants [128]. The improved blood circulation in the endometrium and cervical mucus fertility, decreased hyperandrogenism and insulin resistance, and finally an effect on prostaglandins synthesis and steroidgenesis are the advantages of antioxidant therapy on female fertility [128]. Antioxidants are able to prevent oxidative stress development by either intercepting its formation via termination of propagative oxidative chain reaction or by scavenging excess ROS, therewith maintaining the delicate pro-oxidant/anti-oxidant balance and therefore protecting the cell and microenvironment from oxidative detriment [129]. In an ART setting, antioxidant can be applied to minimize the harmful impacts of endogenous and exogenous sources of ROS on gametes and embryos [129]. Two general treatment approaches were used for applying antioxidant, either as oral supplementations for the subfertile couples several months before to their ART cycle, or as an extra element added to culture media during the ART protocol [129]. There are two varieties of antioxidant systems include enzymes such as superoxide dismutase (SOD), catalase and glutathione peroxidase/reductase, and non-enzymes such as vitamins (E, C, B complex), polyphenols (flavonoids), carotenoids and trace minerals among others [129]. The several previous studies have compared oral antioxidants including: myo-inositol and D-chiro-inositol, N-acetyl-cysteine, melatonin, L-arginine and carnitine, selenium, vitamins E, C and B complex, vitamin D+ calcium, CoQ10, pentoxifylline, and omega-3-polyunsaturzted fatty acids versus placebo, no treatment or standard treatment/another antioxidant [130]. In this section, we specially reviewed the studies that have been performed in PCOS patients.

7.1.1. Myo-Inositol (MYO) and D-Chiro-Inositol (DCI)

Inositol (cyclohexanehexol) is a carbocyclic sugar that has nine stereoisomers, which is commonly referred to as the B vitamin group. Among these inositol, MYO and DCI are known as insulin-sensitizing agents. In addition, inositol acts as an antioxidant that diminish oxidative damage stress by scavenging free radicals [131]. The beneficial effects of MYO are expressed at the ovarian and nonovarian levels and it is an important component of the follicular microenvironment that contributes to both nuclear and cytoplasmatic oocyte development [132]. DCI activity is better expressed in non-ovarian tissues where it may significantly prevent the negative cellular consequences of hyperinsulinemia [133]. Inositol is available in tablet and powder forms which are administrated at doses of 2 to 4 grams per day [134]; however the literature provides no clear data on the appropriate therapeutic dose nor on related adverse effects [131]. Inositol can be prescribed as Inofolic®, a supplement that contains 2 gr of MYO and 200 μgr of folic acid [135].

Interest in inositol as a novel treatment for PCOS was increased following publishing the results of an randomized clinical trial (RCT) that showed DCI markedly improved insulin sensitivity, reduced testosterone, and improved ovulation rates [48]; however, two systematic reviews reported that there were no clear-cut, convincing, evidence based data that confirmed the efficacy of inositol as a treatment for PCOS [131, 136].

Previous studies compared inositol (MYO or DCI) versus placebo, no treatment, or a routine drug (folic acid < 1 mg); inositol (MYO) versus an antioxidant (melatonin); MYO versus an insulin-sensitizing agent (metformin); MYO versus an ovulation induction agent (clomiphene citrate); and inositol (MYO) versus another inositol (DCI) [131]. Two meta-analyses of RCTs published in 2018 reported conflicting results. Pundir et al. evaluated 10 randomized trials of 362 PCOS women treated with MYO and DCI supplements. They concluded that administration of inositol was associated with menstrual cycles regulation and improvements in metabolic parameters; however, evidence was lacking for improvements in pregnancy, miscarriage or live birth [136], therefore a well-designed multicenter trial is required to provide robust evidence of benefit in terms of this issue. Showell et al. evaluated 13 trials that included 1472 subfertile women with PCOS who received myo-inositol as a pre-treatment to IVF. They concluded that there was very low quality evidence in terms of the effect of MYO on live birth or clinical pregnancy rates in subfertile PCOS women pretreated with MYO before IVF compared to standard treatment [131]. In addition, they reported that there was no pooled evidence for administration of MYO versus placebo, another antioxidant, insulin-sensitizing agents, ovulation induction agents, or another type of inositol for PCOS women as pretreatments for IVF and ovulation induction [131].

In 2019, Januszewski et al. conducted a prospective clinical study that evaluated 70 PCOS patients who received combined therapy of a 10:1 ratio of MYO and DCI in the form of one 500 mg inositol tablet, which was administered twice per day for six months [137]. According to the results, this treatment strategy was associated with a statistically significant reduction in body weight and fT, FSH, LH and insulin levels, as well as increased serum SHBG. In addition, serum glucose levels during OGTT decreased after six months of treatment and skin conditions improved after only three months. They concluded that the 10:1 ratio MI and DCI could efficiently improve both metabolic and hormonal parameters in patients with PCOS [138]. Lagana et al. (2018) reported that a 40:1 ratio of MYO:DCI was an appropriate strategy to improve fertility outcomes and extra of DCI might have a detrimental impact on oocyte development [139]. In terms of fertility outcome, Akbari et al. (2019) evaluated 50 infertile PCOS patients in a RCT. The study group patients received daily doses of 4 gr MYO combined with 400 mg folic acid and the control group received 400 mg folic acid from one month prior to the antagonist cycle until the day of ovum pick up [140]. The gene expressions of PGK1, RGS2 and CDC42, which are indicators of oocyte quality in GCs, as well as TAC and ROS levels in follicular fluid were also assessed [140]. The data analysis showed that the metaphase II (MII) oocyte and fertilization rates as well as embryo quality significantly improved in the study group. However, the number of retrieved oocytes and follicle count were not statistically different between groups. PGK1, RGS2 and CDC42 had significantly higher expressions in the study group, but there were no significant differences between the two groups in terms of TAC and ROS levels. They concluded that MYO could alter gene expressions in GCs and improve oocyte and embryo quality among PCOS patients undergoing ART [140].

Finally, the results from the International Consensus Conference on MYO and DCI Inositol in Obstetrics and Gynecology indicated that MYO supplementation at 2g twice per day was more advantageous as PCOS treatment and for prevention of gestational diabetes mellitus [141]. Inositol improved ovarian stimulation parameters in ART and is an attractive treatment option for PCOS; however, available data that pertain to fertility outcomes are conflicting and well-designed clinical trials are warranted to evaluate its effect on spontaneous and non-spontaneous pregnancy and live birth rates [139].

7.1.2. Melatonin

Melatonin (N-acetyl-5-methoxytrypamine), due to its strong antioxidant property, is under consideration as a new agent for PCOS treatment [142]. It is hypothesized that melatonin treatment may significantly assist to maintain the level of gonadal androgens and LH/FSH balance to control PCOS development via MT1 and MT2 receptor proteins [143, 144]. In addition, melatonin can effectively regulate LH receptor gene expression and gonadotropin releasing hormone receptor gene expression in human granulosa lutein cells via the mitogen-activated protein kinase (MAPK) pathway [144, 145]. PCOS women have significantly lower melatonin levels in their follicular fluid than healthy women, and this is related to their ovulatory dysfunction [146]. Administration of melatonin can compensate for this lowered hormone level in follicular fluid and eliminate ovarian dysfunction [142]. The results of melatonin treatment of PCOS patients demonstrated significant impacts on reduced BMI and intra-abdominal fat [142]. Higher melatonin levels in the preovulatory follicles can protect GCs from free radical damage and ultimately prevents the development of PCOS by improving the oocyte quality [144].

To the best of our knowledge, a few studies investigated effect of melatonin on fertility in PCOS patients. The results of some previous studies showed the positive effect of 3 mg melatonin from the fifth day of the previous menstrual cycle until the day of oocyte retrieval in infertile women with prior failure in an IVF cycle [147] or in patients with insomnia who underwent IVF/embryo transfer (ET) cycle [148], and in women with primary infertility who underwent IVF [149]. These studies reported improved fertilization rates [147], oocyte quality [147-149] and higher number of top quality embryos [148, 149], along with a non-significant higher tendency for clinical pregnancy rate [149] with administration of melatonin in ART cycles in non-PCOS patients. One of the most important studies evaluated 40 PCOS patients with normal BMI who received melatonin for six months. The authors noted an association with improvements in androgens and AMH levels and menstrual cycle regularity [150]. On the basis our knowledge, there were two ongoing clinical trials registered at http://clinicaltiral.gov that investigating melatonin treatment in adolescents (NCT00988078) and women diagnosed with PCOS (NCT02663570).

It is proposed that IR of ovarian GCs and overexpression of vascular endothelial growth factor (VEGF) due to insulin stimulation are the underlying mechanisms for poor clinical outcomes in PCOS patients who undergo ART and melatonin may have a positive effect on the ovarian microenvironment by improving IR [142]. Recently, Pacchiarotti et al. [151] conducted a randomized double-blind trial that evaluated 526 PCOS patients who underwent IVF cycle and allocated to three study groups. Participants in group A received Inofolic® plus a daily dose of 4000 mg MYO, 400 mcg folic acid, and 3 mg melatonin. Group B received Inofolic®, a daily dose of 4000 mg MYO and 400 mcg folic acid) and patients in group C (control) only received 400 mcg folic acid. The interventions lasted from the first day of each patient's cycle until 14 days after ET. The results showed that administration of melatonin with MYO significantly enhanced the oocyte and embryo quality, and these supplements had a synergistic effect [151].

Based on the reported evidence, melatonin appears to positively affect metabolic functions in PCOS patients. Some prospective clinical trials reported that melatonin treatment in infertile patients may enhance oocyte and embryo quality, increase the number of mature oocytes, reduce obesity, and ameliorate the proinflammatory state that underlies the development of IR [142]. However, these studies provided low quality evidence on the examined parameters; therefore, clinical trials with larger sample sizes are required to validate the preliminary results that suggest melatonin can be an adjuvant supplementation in ART cycles [152].

7.1.3. N-Acetyl Cysteine (NAC)

NAC is an acetylated variant of the amino acid L-cysteine. Once absorbed, this mucolytic drug metabolizes to cysteine (a precursor of GSH) [153]. NAC can act as insulin sensitize, the antioxidant and anti-inflammatory agent that improves dyslipidemia and IR in PCOS women [153, 154]. Interestingly, Oner et al. conducted a prospective study and concluded that metformin and NAC appear to have similar effects on HA, hyperinsulinaemia and menstrual irregularity in PCOS women [155].

Recently, it has been proposed that antioxidants such as N-acetylcysteine may improve ovarian function and structure through reducing OS in PCOS patients [156]. Saha et al., reviewed the role of NAC in CC-resistant PCOS. They found contradictory results and suggested that more RCTs should be conducted to establish the definitive effect of NAC as an infertility treatment for CC-resistant PCOS [157]:. In the following, Mostajeran et al., in a placebo-controlled double-blind RCT, evaluated the effect of NAC (1.2 g per day) plus letrozole 5 mg per day beginning the third day of menstruation. Their results revealed that NAC was a safe, well-tolerated adjuvant to letrozole and could increase pregnancy rates in PCOS patients [158]. Furthermore, Devi et al. conducted a meta-analysis of 15 RCTs that recruited 2330 females who received NAC as adjuvant therapy for infertility. The data showed that NAC could be an effective adjuvant in PCOS related and unexplained female infertility. The beneficial effects could be more preferred in women with high BMI, IR, and OS. They suggested that more well-designed RCTs with longer follow-up periods should be conducted to examine clinical outcomes such as live birth rate [159]. Thakker et al., in a meta-analysis of eight RCT that included 910 PCOS women demonstrated that NAC significantly improved spontaneous ovulation and live birth rates compared to the placebo [160]. Therefore, based on these studies, there is low to moderate quality evidence to support adjuvant therapy with NAC in ovulation induction with CC or letrozole in PCOS patients; however, further multicenter RCTs are needed to clarify its efficacy on pregnancy and live birth rates.

Elgindy et al., (2010) conducted a preliminary study about the use NAC in ART cycles and concluded that the administration of 1200mg NAC supplementation was not associated with significantly improvements in the numbers of top quality embryos or fertilization and pregnancy rates in ICSI cycles that used the long agonist protocol. However, they proposed that further RCTs that assessed higher doses and/or longer duration of NAC supplementation should be conducted to clarify any significant effects of NAC [161]. In this regard, Cheraghi et al. examined the effect of MET plus NAC during IVF/ICSI treatment in a placebo-controlled RCT that included 80 infertile PCOS patients who were allocated to four study groups: (1) a placebo-treated group that received oral rehydration solution three times per day (TDS); (2) MET-treated group that received MET (500 mg, TDS); (3) NAC-treated group that received NAC (600 mg, TDS); and (4) a group treated with a combination of the same doses of MET plus NAC for a period of six weeks prior to IVF/ICSI cycle [162]. Their findings revealed that the NAC–treated group had a significant decrease in the number of immature and abnormal oocytes and a concomitant increase in the number of good-quality embryos compared with the placebo group. Moreover, there were significant reductions in insulin and LH levels in the MET and NAC groups compared with the placebo-treated group [162]. They concluded that NAC enhanced oocyte and embryo quality and could be considered as an alternative to metformin [162]. However, additional investigation is needed because it is too early to draw any definite conclusions for NAC as an alternative to metformin.

7.1.4. L-Carnitine

L-carnitine is a small water-soluble molecule considered essential for the normal mitochondrial oxidation of long-chain fatty acids and excretion of acyl-coenzyme A (acyl-CoA) esters and it affects adenosine triphosphate (ATP) levels [163, 164]. In 1905, free carnitine was initially isolated from bovine muscle, and it was found that only the L-isomer is bioactive [165, 2]. L-carnitine can protect against free oxygen radical damage to cell membrane and DNA [164]. Moreover, the antioxidant activity of L-carnitine combines the properties of free radical-scavenging and metal-chelating [166]. Abdelrazik et al. initially reported that L-carnitine supplementation in culture media significantly improved embryo quality and blastocyst development rate, and this might provide a novel approach for improving ICSI outcomes in infertile couples [164]. They assumed that the improvement in embryo developmental competence might be related to its potent antioxidant effect and ability to reduce DNA damage, and provide protection for cells from the harmful effects of TNFα [164]. Subsequently, several trials investigated the efficacy of L-carnitine administration on markers of inflammation and indicators of OS; however, their findings were contradictory. In 2018, Maleki et al. conducted a systematic review of six articles to determine the effects of L-carnitine on metabolic variables in PCOS patients [138]. They concluded that an association existed between L-carnitine and improved weight loss, glycemic status and OS. However, further studies should explore the exact mechanisms of the role of L-carnitine role in the treatment of PCOS women [138]. An effective dose of 250 mg L-carnitine per day for 12 weeks was reported in two clinical trials of PCOS patients [167, 168]. The results of these two RCTs showed significant reductions in weight and BMI, waist circumference, FPG, insulin, HOMA-IR and DHEAS [168] as well as improvements of TAC, MDA and MDA/TAC ratio [167]. Recently, Fathizadeh et al. reviewed all scientific databases from 1990 up to May 2020 to determine the effects of L-carnitine supplementation on inflammatory markers and OS. They included 44 studies in this meta-analysis and concluded that an association existed between L-carnitine supplementation and decreased CRP, IL-6, TNF-α, and MDA levels, and increased SOD levels. However, some other inflammatory and OS biomarkers were not affected [169].

Recent evidence has shown that L-carnitine plays important roles in vitro in oocyte growth, oocyte maturation, and embryo development; however, these benefits beneficial have yet to be under-investigated in vivo. To the best of our knowledge, there is one published RCT [170] and a before-after experimental study that have assessed the use of an oral supplement of L-carnitine during ART cycles [141]. Ismail et al. evaluated 170 women diagnosed with PCOS who were resistant to induction ovulation with clomiphene. The patients in the intervention group received 250 mg CC from days 3 until 7 of the cycle in addition to 3 g per day of L-carnitine; while patients in the control group received same induction ovulation protocol plus placebo. Their results demonstrated that the addition of L-carnitine during induction ovulation in CC-resistant PCOS patients not only improved the ovulation quality and pregnancy rate, but also enhanced the patients' lipid profiles and BMI, and had acceptable patient tolerability [170]. In this regard, Kitano et al., in an experimental study, evaluated 214 patients who failed to conceive in previous IVF/ET cycles. All patients received 1000 mg L-carnitine per day for 82 days on average [141]. They observed enhanced embryos quality on days 3 and 5 after insemination following L-carnitine administration compared to previous cycles. It was suggested that oral administration of L-carnitine in infertile women could improve the developmental competence of their oocytes after insemination and result in healthy neonates [141]. There is currently no conclusive evidence to determine whether oral administration of L-carnitine improves ART cycle outcomes in PCOS patients, and well-designed RCTs are warranted in this regard.

7.1.5. Coenzyme Q10 (CoQ10)

CoQ10 is a vitamin-like lipid-soluble substance that acts as an antioxidant agent and it prevents lipid peroxidation and DNA oxidation, as well as empowers the body's energy cycle through ATP production [171, 172]. The results of several studies showed positive effects of CoQ10 on spermatozoa concentration, motility and fertilization rates in cases of male infertility [129]. In 2020, Florou et al. conducted a systematic review and meta-analysis of five RCTs that pertained to CoQ10 therapy on fertility outcomes in women undergoing ART cycles. The study groups comprised 449 infertile women, 215 in the CoQ10 group, and 234 in the placebo/no treatment group [171]. Different treatment doses were reported and included: 600 mg from day 3 of the following menstrual cycle until 8 weeks [173, 174], or 1200 mg from the beginning of the following menstrual cycle until 12 weeks [175] and elsewhere 180 mg from 2nd cycle day until hCG administration day [176, 177]. Their findings demonstrated that an association between oral supplementation of CoQ10 and increased clinical pregnancy rate compared with placebo or no-treatment (OR 2.44, 95% CI 1.30–4.59, p = 0.006). This positive effect remained significant when they separately analyzed women with poor ovarian response and PCOS. They concluded that this adjuvant therapy may improve CPR when compared with placebo or no-treatment without any effect on miscarriage and live birth rates in infertile women who underwent ART cycle [171]. Liu et al., in 2020, published a protocol for a systematic review and meta-analysis to evaluate the effects of CoQ10 supplementation on glucose metabolism, lipid profiles, and biomarkers of inflammation in PCOS women [178]. Samimi et al. also reported that CoQ10 (100 mg per day) for 12 weeks in patients with PCOS resulted in significant reductions in fasting plasma glucose and serum insulin concentrations [179]. Furthermore, Abdulameer Yahya et al. evaluated 41 PCOS patients with hypovitaminosis D in a RCT. They reported that both supplements resulted in significantly decreased free testosterone, LH, LH: FSH ratio, and AMH, in addition to an improvement in the induction ovulation outcome. There was no difference in ovulation rate and CPR when CoQ10 was compared with vitamin D [180]. Elsewhere, Al-Qadhi et al. in a prospective study, assessed 80 PCOS patients in two treatment groups. In the first group, the patients received CoQ10 soft gel capsules 200 mg once per day plus metformin 850 mg twice per day and patients in the control group received metformin only for three consecutive months. The results showed that both treatments were effective on body weight, serum testosterone and OS markers; however, improvements in the CoQ10-metformin group were more significant than the metformin group [181]. Izadi et al. studied the effects of CoQ10 and/or vitamin E on glucose homeostasis parameters and reproductive hormones in 86 PCOS women via a double-blind, placebo-controlled clinical trial. In this trial, CoQ10 supplementation with or without vitamin E for three months in PCOS women had advantageous effects on serum FBS, insulin, HOMA-IR, and total testosterone levels [182]. Based on the above mentioned studies, there are benefits for CoQ10 supplementation on hormonal parameters in PCOS patients. However, few studies have assessed the effect of administration of CoQ10 supplements during ART cycles on pregnancy outcomes in PCOS patients, therefore more RCTs with placebo design are required to reach a better conclusion for this subject.

7.1.6. Vitamin E

Vitamin E is a naturally-occurring, lipid-soluble antioxidant and it is the most active form of alpha-tocopherol that suppresses hydrogen peroxide, superoxide anion, hydroxyl anions and breaks the peroxidation chain reactions [129]. Most research has examined the effect of oral supplementation of vitamin E during ART cycles in infertile male patients. The beneficial effects of this vitamin on sperm motility and function, as well as improved fertilization and pregnancy rates have been observed [129, 183, 184]. There is a consensus in the literature that vitamin E had an important role in ovarian and reproductive physiology because of its ability to protect ovaries from ROS during luteolysis [185]. Riley and Behrman in a review study, reported the beneficial effects of vitamin E and C, as powerful antioxidants, on oocyte maturation, ovulation function, and the uterine environment in animal and human models [186, 187]. Morsy et al., in 2020, conducted a randomized controlled open-label study that evaluated the effect of vitamin E supplementation on fertility outcomes in CC-resistant PCOS patients [187]. The patients were randomly allocated into a control group (n = 30) that received metformin 500 mg three times per day daily to 150 mg CC per day for five days starting from day 3 of menstruation for three menstruation cycles, and the intervention group (n = 30) that received vitamin E 1500 IU per day for the entire study period plus metformin and CC according to the same previous regimen. The results demonstrated that vitamin E did not increase the ovulation and pregnancy rates in women with CC-resistant PCOS. Fatemi et al. also conducted a double-blinded RCT that evaluated 105 infertile PCOS women who underwent ICSI cycles. The patients were divided into a treatment group (n =52) that received vitamin E 400 mg per day and vitamin D3 50000 IU/once per two weeks then 3300 IU per day or a placebo group (n = 53) for eight weeks [188]. The results showed that combined supplementation of vitamin E plus vitamin D3 for eight weeks along with dietary counseling significantly improves clinical pregnancy in PCOS women treated with IVF/ICSI; however, these improvements were observed without an increase in the TAC level or reduced oxidative factors [188]. Therefore, their findings did not support the hypothesis that vitamins E and D3 might play a role in the success rate of

IVF via an antioxidant mechanism. Further trials that have two separate groups for vitamin D3 and vitamin E are warranted to better understand the role of each micronutrient in increasing implantation and pregnancy rates [188].

Cicek et al., in a prospective non-randomized study on women with unexplained infertility, reported that vitamin E enhanced the endometrial environment, which was possibly due to its antioxidant and anticoagulant effects, and by modulation of the anti-estrogenic effect of CC; however, no effect on implantation or pregnancy rates were observed [189]. Presumably, the role of vitamin E in improving endometrial thickness may be due to its anticoagulation property which is associated with increased blood flow to follicles and granulating cells. This subsequently produced sufficient amounts of estrogen led to proper endometrial preparation for better implantation [188, 189]. There is little evidence in this area, and more RCTs are needed for accurate conclusions.

7.1.7. Vitamin C

Vitamin C (L –ascorbic acid) is a water-soluble, chain-breaking antioxidant. Previous studies demonstrated that vitamin C concentrations are lower in PCOS patients than in controls [96]. Several vitamins with antioxidant capacities derived from their scavenging of oxidant molecules have been studied in PCOS [190], but the studies in the case of vitamin C are limited.

Its use as adjuvant therapy in female infertility was assessed by Griesinger et al., in a large double-blind RCT. They evaluated vitamin C supplements (1-10 gr) that were administered for 14 days beginning on the ovum pick-up day in women who underwent IVF/ET. Their results showed no difference in implantation and clinical pregnancy rates between the vitamin C and placebo groups [191]. However, Henmi et al. in a prospective randomized study, assessed oral vitamin C supplementation (750 mg) that started on the first day of the third menstrual cycle until a positive urine pregnancy test (maximum six months) in infertile women with luteal phase defects who were not on IVF/ET. The control group received no treatment. Their findings demonstrated that oral vitamin C supplementation was associated with significantly increased progesterone levels and clinical pregnancy rates [192].

Based on our knowledge, there is scant evidence regarding vitamin C supplementation on fertility outcomes in PCOS women. Forouhar et al. conducted a double-blinded RCT that evaluated the effectiveness of vitamin C in a balanced diet for two months on the levels of related hormones in infertile PCOS women. The results showed no significant effect of vitamin C in comparison to a placebo group in terms of serum FSH, testosterone, progesterone, and estradiol levels after two months of intervention. Elsewhere, Panti et al. in a single-blind RCT compared the effect of antioxidant supplementation Vitacap®, which contains vitamins A, B1, C, B_6, B_{12}, D_3, and minerals, with placebo on fertility outcomes in women with PCOS. All participants underwent ovulation induction with CC and were followed for six months. The findings showed a statistically significance difference in the serum levels of OS marker and antioxidant enzymes between the two groups. Interestingly, the clinical pregnancy and live birth rates in the antioxidant therapy group were significantly higher than the placebo group [193]. The results of this trial were in contrast to recent Cochrane review by Showell et al. (2020) that found very low-quality evidence to suggest antioxidant may be associated with increased rates of clinical pregnancy or live birth [130]. Therefore, the authors suggested that larger multicenter RCTs should be conducted to confirm the conclusion of this review article.

7.1.8. Vitamin D

Vitamin D3 (cholecalciferol), the sunshine vitamin, is obtained from fish oils or produced by the skin from 7-dehydrocholesterol after exposure to ultraviolet irradiation [194]. Its receptors are expressed in 2776 genomic positions and it regulates the expression of 229 genes in more than 30 different tissues, including the ovaries [195, 196]. Vitamin D may contribute in glucose metabolism by increasing insulin synthesis and release, and increasing insulin receptor expression or suppression of proinflammatory cytokines that are possibly involved in the development of IR [197]. Therefore, the impact of vitamin D on metabolic and reproductive dysfunctions in PCOS may be mediated by IR [196]. The results of some studies show that PCOS might also be at increased risk of vitamin D deficiency (VDD) [196]. Straight associations of VDD with some approved comorbidities of PCOS such as type 2 diabetes, IR, metabolic syndrome, and cardiovascular diseases have been reported [198-201]. In a recent systematic and meta-analysis, He et al. [196] evaluated 30 studies that pertained to PCOS and vitamin D levels. They found an association with lower serum vitamin D levels and metabolic and hormonal disorders in women with PCOS. Specifically, PCOS patients with VDD were more prone to increased levels of FBS and HOMA-IR index compared to those without VDD. However, this meta-analysis did not find any evidence to support that vitamin D supplementation could reduce or relieve metabolic and hormonal dysfunctions in PCOS. They mentioned that VDD might be a comorbid manifestation of PCOS or a minor pathway in PCOS associated metabolic and hormonal dysfunctions [196]. Therefore, they suggested stronger prospective and RCTs that had repeated VDD assessments and better characterization of PCOS phenotypes at enrollment would be needed to clarify the role of VDD, either as a co-determinant or a consequence of hormonal and metabolic dysregulations in PCOS [196].

Recently several review articles and meta-analyses have been published related to the effect of Vitamin D3 supplementation in ART cycles [202-204]. In 2018, Chu et al. concluded that women who undergo ART cycles and have sufficient vitamin D levels are associated with higher live birth rates than women who have vitamin D deficiency or insufficiency [202]. They mentioned that a large multicenter RCT should be conducted to study the benefits of treatment VDD to test this hypothesis [202]. In contrast, Cozzolino et al. reported that serum vitamin D levels did not influence IVF outcomes in terms of clinical pregnancy, live birth, and miscarriage rates [204]. A protocol of a RCT, the "SUNDRO study, was published by Paffoni et al. who investigated the effect of vitamin D supplementation on ART outcome [205]. The results of this study could help resolve the controversies regarding vitamin D supplementation in women who undergo ART cycles. There is limited data especially addressed the role of Vitamin D in women with PCOS who undergo IVF/ICSI cycles. Although, Orman et al., in 2020, reported a positive correlation between serum vitamin D and the number of retrieved oocytes and fertilization rate in women with PCOS [206], they found no correlation between vitamin D levels and clinical pregnancy rate. Dastorani et al. in a RCT compared the effect of vitamin D supplementation (50000 IU per week) with a placebo group (n=20) for eight weeks in 40 infertile women 18–40 years of age, who were diagnosed with PCOS and were candidates for IVF. They concluded that vitamin D supplementation had beneficial effects on insulin metabolism and the lipid profiles of infertile PCOS patients; however, they did not report a comparison of IVF outcomes between groups the two groups [207]. To the best of our knowledge, there is no evidence that vitamin D supplementation can improve fertility outcomes for women with PCOS who are candidates for IVF, and further studies in this area are suggested.

7.1.9. Selenium (Se)

Se is an exceptional essential trace element that has several important functions at the cellular level and organism in animal and human health [208]. The biological functions of Se are carried out by selenoproteins [208] that act as ROS degrading selenoenzymes that have antioxidant and anti-inflammatory effects [209]. Selenoproteins are related to important cellular processes such as synthesis of desoxynucleotides for DNA, scavenging of harmful signaling peroxides, depletion of oxidized proteins and membranes, redox signaling control, metabolism of thyroid hormones, and protein folding [208, 210]. The exact underlying molecular and biochemical mechanisms by which Se or selenoproteins modulate female reproduction are mostly unclear [208].

The addition of sodium selenite (2.5 and 25 ng/mL) to the culture medium in the animal model has been reported in improving the developmental competence, the blastocyst rate, and overall quality of embryos by limiting the oxidative injury and programmed cell death [208]. Two recent clinical studies evaluated the effect of Se supplementation as a micronutrient supplement on IVF outcomes where they administered Se supplementation at doses of 50 or 27.5 µg for three or two months prior to ovarian puncture to infertile women undergoing IVF/ICSI cycle [211]. The results showed an association between Se supplementation and a significant increase in the mean number of good quality oocytes [211] as well as significant improvements in embryonic quality [212]. The limitations of these studies included an underpowered design, very small sample sizes and Se supplementation that was administered in combination with other micronutrients [208]. However, these findings could be a useful foundation for researchers to design powerful clinical trials that could demonstrate the importance of these micronutrients for women who undergo IVF.

Recently, Atef et al. reported the therapeutic potential of sodium selenite in a letrozole induced PCOS rat model. The authors concluded that Se treatment of these PCOS rats was successful and comparable to metformin [213]. In addition, treatment with Se was associated with significant improvements in PCOS related endocrine and metabolic phenotypes and histopathological changes via modulation of mitochondrial dynamics, anti-apoptotic action, reduction of OS and mitochondrial dysfunction. Therefore, it was suggested that Se could provide a novel therapeutic strategy for PCOS [213]. Heidar et al., in 2019, randomly allocated 36 women with PCOS who were candidates into an intervention group that received 200 µg per day of Se or a placebo group for eight weeks. The results showed that Se supplementation significantly downregulated gene expressions of IL-1 and TNF-α in addition to significant upregulation of vascular VEGF gene expression in lymphocytes of PCOS patients in the intervention group compared with the placebo group [214]. Overall, the authors concluded that Se supplementation for eight weeks could improve IL-1, TNF-α, and VEGF gene expressions in infertile PCOS women undergoing IVF, but it had no impact on clinical symptoms and gene expressions of TGF-β and IL-8. Jamilian et al. reported that Se and probiotic co-supplementation for 12 weeks in women with PCOS was associated with significant reductions in total testosterone, hirsutism, OS and a few biomarkers of inflammation [215]. In addition, Köse et al. demonstrated that Se significantly alleviated OS via transient receptor potential cation channel subfamily V member 1 channels in the neutrophils of patients with PCOS [216].

According to the recent review article in this regard, there is low quality evidence for support use of Se supplementation in men and women who seek fertility treatment [217]. Additional well-designed, randomized, controlled trials are warranted that could ascertain the effect of Se supplementation on fertility outcomes in infertile women, in particular, those diagnosed with PCOS.

7.1.10. Quercetin

Quercetin is a bioactive flavonoid found in more than 100 types of Chinese herbs, [218] which has radical scavenging and antioxidant properties and is extensively used to treat metabolic and inflammatory disorders [219]. Most fruits and vegetables, particularly onions, apples, berries, citrus, red grapes, nuts, seeds and tea are good sources of quercetin [220]. Quercetin is an active ingredient in hawthorn that has therapeutic effects against inflammation, diabetes, and their complications [218]. The results of several pharmacological have shown that quercetin supplements are effective in the modulation of redux status [221], alleviation of inflammation [222], inhibition of platelet aggregation [223], relax vessels smooth muscles [224], and prevention of LDL oxidation [225], hypertension [226], and diabetes [227]. The hypoglycemic impact of quercetin may be related to insulin signal transduction, such as increased protein expression, and tyrosine phosphorylation of the insulin receptor, and several insulin receptor substrates (IRSs) and glucose transporters (GLUTs) [228]. Moreover, quercetin exerts an insulin-sensitizing effect by promoting the proliferation of pancreatic β-cells and enhancing glucose metabolism and insulin secretion [229]. The ability of quercetin to inhibit xanthine oxidase via reduction of free radicals production, modulation of antioxidants and prevention of lipid peroxidation has prompted researchers to consider it as antioxidant agent [230].

According to a recent systematic review, five studies in animal PCOS models and three clinical trials were performed to evaluate the therapeutic effect of quercetin on PCOS [231]. The ovarian morphology, weight and diameter were investigated in five of eight studies. The results of these studies demonstrated significant improvements in ovarian morphology, folliculogenesis, and luteinization [218, 232-235] as well as decreases in ovarian diameter and cystic follicle diameter after quercetin therapy [232].

Generally, the findings showed significantly increased normal follicles in ovaries, restored normal ovarian anatomy, and improvements in uterine histology after treatment that were comparable to metformin [232-235]. Five of eight studies evaluated the impacts of quercetin on reproductive hormones in PCOS subjects [232, 236, 237]. The results of these studies demonstrated improved in menstrual cyclicity [218, 234], reductions in testosterone, LH, and estradiol levels [232, 234, 236, 237] in addition to improvement in subsiding hirsutism [232, 234]. Jahan et al. reported that quercetin could regulate steroidogenesis via decreasing testosterone levels and improving progesterone and estradiol levels. In these studies, patients had significant decrease in the insulin and glucose levels, and HOMA-IR after administration of quercetin intake [218, 233, 234, 236]. Quercetin at a dose of 25 mg/kg was associated with a significant decrease in plasma glucose levels in PCOS rats [235]. Rezvan et al. reported that oral quercetin supplementation enhanced the serum levels of total adiponectin by 5.56% and high-molecular-weight (HMW) adiponectin by 3.9% in PCOS women compared to a placebo group [238]. Moreover, the impressive role of quercetin in improving adiponectin-mediated IR and the hormonal profile of women with PCOS was shown [231]. To the best of our knowledge, studies have been conducted to investigate the effect of quercetin on oocyte quality in the animal model, and no studies have been found in PCO infertile women, and researches in this area is recommended.

7.2. Adjunctive Anti-Inflammatory Therapy

PCOS could be considered as a chronic pro-inflammatory state because of the increase in some pro-inflammatory cytokines levels in the peripheral circulation of PCOS patients [156]; however, whether altered inflammatory cytokines expression in PCOS patients is associated with a resistant response to CC is unclear [239]. Wang et al. conducted a cross-sectional study and reported that altered angiopoietin-2 and CXCL-16 levels might compromise the responsiveness of the ovaries to CC via up-regulation of angiogenesis and inflammation [239]. We particularly reviewed the published studies concerning that several drugs with anti-inflammatory effects were evaluated as adjuvant therapy to improve fertility outcomes in PCOS patients.

7.2.1. Metformin

Metformin is a biguanide that is used to reduce blood sugar level. It has limited side effects and is a first line treatment in patients who suffer from type II diabetes mellitus [240]. Hasanpour et al., reviewed several studies and confirmed the anti-inflammatory and antioxidant roles of metformin that occur via with multiple mechanisms. Activation of AMPK by metformin has had a clue role in many of them [240]. Metformin is one of the earliest drugs used to treat PCOS and many studies have been conducted due to its direct effects on glucose metabolism [241] and human ovarian steroidogenesis [242]. Significant improvements in insulin sensitivity and anthropometric parameters in PCOS women have been observed with different administration doses ranged from 500mg to 2550mg (850mg tid) [126]. Based on recent international evidence–based guidelines, metformin along with lifestyle modification could be considered in adolescents and adult PCOS women for weight control, and hormonal and metabolic outcomes [243]. In our opinion, administration of metformin in infertile women with the syndrome is so well established that many studies use metformin as a routine or control treatment to compare the experimental drugs. Morley et al., in a Cochrane review article stated that the metformin therapy resulted in higher ovulation, pregnancy and live birth rates compared to placebo in infertile PCOS women; however, the quality of evidence was low to moderate [244]. Therefore, in PCOS women who are CC-resistant, adjuvant therapy with metformin improved ovulation and clinical pregnancy rates, but it was not associated with higher live birth rates [244].

The results of studies that administer metformin prior to or during an ART cycle for women with PCOS are inconsistent. Mourad et al., in a Cochrane review article, reported a moderate quality of evidence for consideration of metformin therapy prior and during an ART cycle in women with PCOS as a preventive strategy for OHSS [244]. limited evidence suggests that reporting metformin may increase live birth rates among subfertile women with PCOS who undergo ovulation induction with gonadotropins along with timed intercourse or intrauterine insemination [245]. In contrast, Kjotrod et al. conducted in a RCT with metformin/placebo therapy for non-obese infertile anovulatory PCOS women undergoing IVF-ET and found no significant effects of metformin on the efficacy of ART per se [246]. According to recent guideline, metformin alone compared with placebo enhanced the ovulation rate in infertile PCOS women; however, it should not be applied as first-line therapy for anovulation because CC or letrozole alone are much more effective in increasing ovulation, pregnancy, and live-birth rates in these women [247]. Recently, Kalem et al. conducted a retrospective study that evaluated the effect of metformin therapy prior to IVF cycles in 96 PCOS women who were between 24 and 40 years of age. They found no beneficial effects of metformin therapy in increasing the treatment success in the IVF/ICSI cycles [248]. In addition, they concluded that it would be appropriate to limit administration of this agent in special indications such as decreasing IR [248]. Similarly, a systematic meta-analysis study conducted by Wu et al. (2020) examined data from 12 RCTs that collectively included 1123 women. They concluded that metformin therapy was associated with a decreased risk of OHSS among women with PCOs who were undergoing IVF, and there was no effect on clinical pregnancy or live birth rates in the total studied population; however, metformin was associated with an increased clinical pregnancy rate among women with BMI values of 26 or greater [249]. Eventually, they suggested that metformin therapy should be carefully considered for PCOS women undergoing IVF and might be more preferred in women with a BMI of 26 or greater [249]. Abu Hashim in a review article, mentioned that there was no evidence for a decreased risk of spontaneous miscarriage or enhanced risk of major anomalies in women with PCOS who received metformin during the first trimester [250]. Although the therapeutic administration of metformin is considered safe, results of recent epidemiological studies indicated phenotypic differences after prenatal exposure to metformin [126]; therefore, we propose that more clinical studies should be conducted to evaluate this issue especially during ART cycles.

7.2.2. Omega-3-Polyunsaturzted Fatty Acids

The antioxidant and anti-inflammatory effects of supplementation with omega-3 suggest an assumptive role in improving insulin sensitivity and lipid profiles of women with PCOS [156]. Omega-3 fatty acids supplements could improve insulin sensitivity by producing and secreting anti-inflammatory adipokines (such as adiponectin) and lowering inflammation and proinflammatory cytokines [251-254]. Recently, Tosatti et al., concluded that supplementation with n-3 fatty acids could reduce the inflammatory state in women with PCOS via a decrease in hs-CRP and an increase in adiponectin levels [255]. Yang et al. (2018), in a systematic review and meta-analysis, evaluated nine RCTs with 591 PCOS patients. The dose (900-4000 mg) and duration of omega-3 fatty acid administration (6-12 weeks) as well as type of co-treatment drug (metformin or vitamin E) in the various studies differed. Their data analysis showed that omega-3 fatty acids may improve the HOMA index, decrease TC and TG levels, and increase adiponectin levels. According to these evidences, the authors concluded that omega-3 fatty acids may be recommended for the treatment of PCOS with evaluated lipid profiles (TC, LDL-C and TG) as well as IR [253]. Mirmasoumi et al. examined the effect of flaxseed oil omega-3 fatty acid supplementation (1000 mg per day) compared to placebo (twice a day) for 12 weeks in 60 PCOS women aged 18–40 years. Overall, the results showed that flaxseed oil omega-3 supplementation had beneficial effects on insulin metabolism, modified Ferriman-Gallwey scores, serum TG, VLDL-cholesterol and hs-CRP levels; however, it had no effect on hormonal and other lipid profiles, and plasma nitric oxide levels [256]. Haidari et al., in an open-label RCT, found that flaxseed supplementation plus lifestyle modification was more effective compared to lifestyle modification alone in all biochemical and anthropometric variables in patients with PCOS [257].

To the best of our knowledge, the use of omega -3 supplementation before and during an IVF therapy has not been assessed in any well-designed randomized prospective study. Based on previous evidences, long-chain omega-3 fatty acids were positively related with improved fertility in both women and men [258]. Recently, Bareksei et al., evaluated the effects of periconceptual omega-3-fatty acid supplementation on IVF success and miscarriage rates in patients of a German fertility center [258]. This study was not entirely prospective and a group of 52 infertile patients with a history of at least two miscarriages or unsuccessful IVF approaches received periconceptional omega-3-fatty acid supplementation for at least three weeks prior to the IVF cycle. The "historical" control group consisted of 1109 patients who did not receive omega-3-fatty acid supplementation and were recruited from the fertility center's patient database. They concluded that omega-3-fatty acid supplementation led to significantly improved IVF success rates as well as a reduction in miscarriage rates compared to patients in the control group. Interestingly, Vahed et al., demonstrated that the addition of omega-3 to the environment of oocyte or cumulus cells affected oocytes and cumulus cells maturation, which was followed by the differential expression of TRIB genes. This findings suggested a role for fatty acid metabolism in differentiation and maturation of cumulus cells [259]. This results encouraged the design of further age-matched, double-blinded prospective studies in order to clarify the exact influence of effect of periconceptional omega-3-fatty acid supplementation on fertility rates [258].

7.2.3. Statins

Statins are pharmacologic agents that selectively inhibit 3-hydroxy-3-methylglutaryl-coenzyme A reductase, the rate-limiting enzyme in the cholesterol biosynthetic pathway [260]. Administration of statins has been evaluated in PCOS obese women with concomitant lipid disorders [156]. In three RCT, reduced serum testosterone levels and improvements in hirsutism after simvastatin treatment of patients with PCOS have been reported [260-262]. Celik and Acbay compared the effects of metformin and metformin plus rosuvastatin on HA in PCOS patients. Their findings demonstrated similar reductions in BMI, insulin, and glucose levels in both groups after 12 weeks of treatment; however, a greater decline was observed in total and free testosterone levels in patients who received the combination therapy. In addition, the DHEA-S levels significantly decreased in patients treated with a combination of metformin and rosuvastatin [263]. According to this evidence, it is proposed that some of the statins may affect ovarian function [260]. Rashidi et al. conducted an RCT that evaluated the effects of simvastatin on androgens, inflammatory mediators, and endogenous pituitary gonadotropins in PCOS women undergoing IVF. In this trial, 64 PCOS patients were randomly allocated into two groups. The patients in the intervention group received 20 mg oral simvastatin (n = 32), whereas patients in the control group received a placebo (n = 29) for eight weeks before initiating their IVF treatment [260].The results indicated that simvastatin might be compatible with gonadotropin therapy for IVF and could offer beneficial endocrine and cardiovascular effects for patients with PCOS who undergo ET. Although the reductions in hsCRP and vascular cell adhesion protein-1 after simvastatin treatment were significant, the observed improvements in reproductive function were mild, therefore, further RCTs were suggested to clarify simvastatin's impact on reproductive physiology [260].

Gao et al. [264], in a meta-analysis, examined the data from four RCTs that administered statins to PCOS patients. After the data analysis, they observed the significant differences in reducing serum total testosterone levels when comparing statins with placebo or statin + metformin with metformin. In addition, statin was more effective than placebo in reducing LDL, TC, and TG levels, as well as the statin plus metformin, was more effective than metformin in lowering LDL. TC, and TG levels. There were some concerns regarding the conclusion of this meta-analysis due to that blinding and concealment were explicitly described in only two studies [265, 266] and both selective and measurement bias could not be determined in the other studies [264]. One of the weaknesses of previous studies was that clinical outcomes that including ovarian function and fertility were not reported in patients [264]. Puurunen et al. (2013) conducted in a double-blind RCT to compare the effect of atorvastatin therapy (20 mg per day) or placebo for six months in 28 PCOS patients. They concluded that atorvastatin therapy improved chronic inflammation and lipid profiles, but it impaired insulin sensitivity in women with PCOS [267].

Sun et al., in a meta-analysis, recently evaluated four RCTs regarding therapeutic effects of statins with metformin on PCOS patients [268]. They found that combined statin and metformin therapy could improve lipid and inflammation parameters; however, it was not effective in improving insulin sensitivity and reducing of HA in PCOS women. They suggested that a large-scale RCT should be conducted to clarify the long-term effects of this therapy. Seyam et al. [269] conducted a double-blind RCT that compared the effectiveness of simvastatin 20 mg per day versus using placebo for six months in young unmarried PCOS women. The results showed that administration of simvastatin was associated with a significant decrease in serum levels of testosterone, LH, and the LH/FSH ratio as well as a clear reduction in TC, LDL, and triglyceride levels compared to placebo. However, no significant difference in IR was found after treatment in both groups. In addition, significant improvements in menstrual regularity and simvastatin alleviated hirsutism, acne, ovarian volume, and BMI in these women. Interestingly, spontaneous ovulation was detected by sonography and measurement of progesterone in 10% of patients in the study group compared to none in the placebo group. They subsequently examined the effects of prolonged statin use on clinical and biochemical abnormalities and ovulation dysfunction in another double-blind RCT in 200 young single women with PCOS. In this trial, the combined use of simvastatin 20 mg per day with metformin 500 mg tid for one year were compared with separated use of simvastatin and metformin as the control groups. The combined simvastatin and metformin treatment showed significant improvements in PCOS clinical and ovarian dysfunction abnormalities that was greater than their individual treatment [270].

The results of several RCT with low sample sizes demonstrated beneficial effects of statins (especially simvastatin) alone or in combination to metformin on ovarian function, chronic inflammation and lipid profile of PCOS women [270, 271]; however, this issue is still being under investigation and more RCTs prior to or during ART cycles are recommended.

7.2.4. Resveratrol

Resveratrol (3,5,4-trihydroxy-transstilbene), a natural polyphenol is found in grasp, berries and peanuts; it is produced in plants as a natural defense mechanism in response to UV, and fungal and bacterial infections

[126]. The anti-inflammatory, antioxidant and cardioprotective actions of resveratrol have been reported [272]. Moreover, some in vitro studies showed the inhibitory effects of resveratrol on proliferation, mevalonate pathway activity and cholesterol synthesis in theca-interstitial cell cultures [273]. Zhu et al., in a recent meta-analysis, evaluated nine RCTs on resveratrol therapy and reported that this natural element might be a beneficial treatment for diabetes mellitus type 2 because of improvements in FBS and insulin levels, and reductions in the HOMA-IR index. According to these evidences, resveratrol is considered a new treatment option for women with PCOS [274]. Banaszewska et al. [275] in a double-blinded RCT investigated the effects of oral resveratrol supplementation 3500 mg for three months in young PCOS patients. They found that this supplementation significantly reduced total testosterone, DHESA and FBS levels in comparison to placebo. The authors reported some adverse effects, which were predominantly nausea, vomiting and diarrhea and liver dysfunction with the oral dose of 1500 mg per day. In addition, Ortega et al. conducted a RCT that evaluated the effect of resveratrol 2gr for nine days for prevention of OHSS in high risk egg donors who were undergoing ovarian stimulation protocols [276]. Their findings showed that prophylactic treatment with resveratrol did not reduce either the incidence of OHSS or the VEGF concentration [276]. Therefore, it is difficult to determine the lowest therapeutic dose of resveratrol is difficult [126]. Recently, Brenjian et al. [277] conducted an RCT that investigated the effect of resveratrol treatment on pro-inflammatory and endoplasmic reticulum stress markers in patients with PCOS. Cumulus cells were obtained from 40 patients with PCOS who were divided into two groups: resveratrol 800 mg per day and placebo for 40 days [277]. They found that serum levels of IL-6, IL-1β, TNF-α, IL-18, NF-κB, and CRP decreased in the treatment group. Furthermore, gene expression analysis demonstrated that the expression levels of ATF4 and ATF6 significantly increased in the resveratrol treatment group, whereas the expression levels of CHOP, GRP78, and XBP1 significantly decreased. The authors concluded that resveratrol has anti-inflammatory effects via the suppression of NF-κB and NF-κB–regulated gene products; moreover, it could modulate endoplasmic reticulum stress in

GCs by altering the expression of genes involved in the unfolding protein response process [277]. To the best of our knowledge, this natural supplement is still under investigation and no study has evaluated resveratrol on fertility outcome in ART or non-ART cycles. Therefore, we suggested that long-term, well-designed RCTs should be conducted to clarify the effectiveness and safety of resveratrol as treatment for PCOS.

7.3. Life Style Modification

Lifestyle modification (LSM) in PCOS patients has been studied for more than a decade. Teede et al., in an international evidence-based guideline, recommended multicomponent lifestyle intervention that included a specific hypocaloric diet, physical exercise and behavioral changes) for all obese or overweight women with PCOS in order to reduction of weight, central obesity and IR according to available moderate quality evidence-based data [243]. A meta-analysis by Kim et al. (2020) combined data from 11 RCTs to evaluate the effectiveness of LSM plus metformin and metformin alone [278]. This meta-analysis showed that no significant difference existed in improvements in the women's menstrual cycles between LSM versus metformin alone and between LSM plus metformin versus LSM [278]. Moreover, LSM was associated with decreased IR as well as increased serum levels of sex hormone-binding globulins compared with metformin alone. The pregnancy rates and body mass indices were similar between LSM and metformin alone. Therefore, they recommended LSM for women with PCOS in cases where metformin is not indicated [278]. Nevertheless, all the studies confirmed fairly similar improvements in the main manifestations of PCOS, even with a significantly moderate weight loss, and specifically on menstrual cyclicity and ovulatory rates, other than on hormonal and metabolic parameters [279, 280].

Available data support the concept that a significant improvement in achieving higher natural ovulation and fertility rates is possible after LSM [280]. The possibility of pregnancy is critically related to the amount of weight loss [280]. It is proposed that a healthy diet can positively affect fertility processes in normal weight PCOS women [280]. Li et al. reported that preconception weight loss with a target goal of ≥ 10% could benefit the patients' clinical outcomes and recommended it for obese women with PCOS prior to ART [281]. However, there is limited, and conflicting data regarding the role of dietary intervention prior to the ART cycle [254, 282, 283]. Alibeigi et al., in a clinical trial, examined the effect of a traditional medicine-oriented diet and lifestyle for three months on IVF outcomes in 180 infertile women diagnosed with ovulatory problems, endometriosis or idiopathic infertility factors [284]. Their results demonstrated that this intervention was associated with a significant increase in the total number of retrieved and MII oocytes, number and quality of obtained embryo, and improvements in fertilization and overall pregnancy rates compared to the control group [284]. A recent, large RCT conducted by Van Oer et al. ascertained the cost-effectiveness of lifestyle intervention that preceded infertility treatment compared to prompt treatment [285]. Infertile obese women (BMI ≥29 kg/m^2) were randomly allocated to a six month lifestyle intervention program prior to infertility treatment (n = 290) or to prompt infertility treatment (n = 287). The live birth rate within 24 months after randomization was considered to be a primary outcome [285]. The result of this trial was discouraging because it was reported that lifestyle intervention in obese infertile women prior to infertility treatment was not associated with higher rates of physiological delivery compared with prompt infertility treatment. Thus this intervention was not a cost-effective strategy in terms of healthy live birth rate [285]. Unfortunately, no similar studies have been carried out in obese PCOS women [280]; therefore, further high-powered clinical studies are recommended for these patients.

Dietary changes are one of the most important components of lifestyle modification. Most previous studies evaluated energy restricted diets in infertile women with PCOS [286, 287]. Recently, an anti-inflammatory diet was proposed as a new dietary strategy. Salama et al., in a prospective clinical trial evaluated the effect of an anti-inflammatory dietary approach with a pharmacological target for management of an overweight and obese PCOS population [288]. The anti-inflammatory approach with low GI foods in a Mediterranean style; reduced red meat and processed meat intake;

prohibited added sugar and lowered saturated fat; encouraged herbs, spices, phytochemicals, antioxidants, and low omega-6 fatty acids and high omega-3 fatty acids intake; small frequent meals; and an achievable form of exercise. Pharmacological agents often act downstream from the true primary molecular target of inflammation, while anti-inflammation nutrition works upstream to decrease the dietary factors that activate NF-kB to generate silent inflammation [288]. The success of this anti-inflammatory diet can be examined clinically by various markers of silent inflammation, which include fibrinogen, CRP, and SAA, and by improvements in conditions with metabolic dysfunction such as type II diabetes mellitus, metabolic syndrome, and cardiovascular disease [288, 289]. The results of this trial showed that this dietary approach was associated with good prognostic metabolic and reproductive responses to weight loss in overweight and obese women with PCOS [288]. These authors in another prospective clinical study, revealed that addition of metformin (850 mg twice per day) to lifestyle modifications (anti-inflammatory diet) was not better than lifestyle modifications alone in terms of menstrual frequency, pregnancy rates, weight loss, reduction of IR, or alleviation of HA [290]. This type of diet is currently being studied alone or in combination with some herbal medicines. The application of any lifestyle intervention in women with PCOS to improve fertility is still a conflicting issue. More studies are needed to determine its efficacy and cost-effectiveness, especially when used during preconception. It should be taken into consideration when designing short and long-term studies. The patients under consideration should not have psychological problems and they must be very committed and responsive to the offered strategies [280].

REFERENCES

[1] Rojas J, Chávez M, Olivar L, Rojas M, Morillo J, Mejías J, et al. Polycystic Ovary Syndrome, Insulin Resistance, and Obesity: Navigating the Pathophysiologic Labyrinth. *International Journal of Reproductive Medicine.* 2014;2014:719050.

[2] El Hayek S, Bitar L, Hamdar LH, Mirza FG, Daoud G. *Poly Cystic Ovarian Syndrome: An Updated Overview*. 2016;7(124).

[3] Wang R, Mol BWJJHR. *The Rotterdam criteria for polycystic ovary syndrome: evidence-based criteria?* 2017;32(2):261-4.

[4] Goldrat O, Delbaere A. PCOS: update and diagnostic approach. 2018.

[5] Kalhori Z, Mehranjani MS, Azadbakht M, Shariatzadeh *MAJR, Fertility, Development. l-Carnitine improves endocrine function and folliculogenesis by reducing inflammation, oxidative stress and apoptosis in mice following induction of polycystic ovary syndrome*. 2019;31(2):282-93.

[6] de Melo AS, Rodrigues JK, Junior AAJ, Ferriani RA, Navarro PAJR. *Oxidative stress and polycystic ovary syndrome: an evaluation during ovarian stimulation for intracytoplasmic sperm injection*. 2017;153(1):97-105.

[7] Morgante G, Massaro M, Di Sabatino A, Cappelli V, De Leo VJGE. *Therapeutic approach for metabolic disorders and infertility in women with PCOS*. 2018;34(1):4-9.

[8] Kelly CC, Lyall H, Petrie JR, Gould GW, Connell JM, Sattar NJTJoCE, et al. *Low grade chronic inflammation in women with polycystic ovarian syndrome*. 2001;86(6):2453-5.

[9] Patel S. Polycystic ovary syndrome (PCOS), an inflammatory, systemic, lifestyle endocrinopathy. *J Steroid Biochem Mol Biol*. 2018;182:27-36.

[10] Hong L, Zhang Y, Wang Q, Han Y, Teng X. Effects of interleukin 6 and tumor necrosis factor-α on the proliferation of porcine theca interna cells: Possible role of these cytokines in the pathogenesis of polycystic ovary syndrome. *Taiwan J Obstet Gynecol*. 2016; 55(2):183-7.

[11] Furat Rencber S, Kurnaz Ozbek S, Eraldemır C, Sezer Z, Kum T, Ceylan S, et al. Effect of resveratrol and metformin on ovarian reserve and ultrastructure in PCOS: an experimental study. *J Ovarian Res*. 2018;11(1):55.

[12] Brouillet S, Boursier G, Anav M, Du Boulet De La Boissière B, Gala A, Ferrieres-Hoa A, et al. *C-reactive protein and ART outcomes: a systematic review.* 2020.

[13] Kahyaoglu S, Yumuşak OH, Ozyer S, Pekcan MK, Erel M, Cicek MN, et al. *Clomiphene citrate treatment cycle outcomes of polycystic ovary syndrome patients based on basal high sensitive C-reactive protein levels: a cross-sectional study.* 2017;10(4):320.

[14] Escobar-Morreale HF, Luque-Ramírez M, González FJF, sterility. *Circulating inflammatory markers in polycystic ovary syndrome: a systematic review and metaanalysis.* 2011;95(3):1048-58. e2.

[15] Borthakur A, Prabhu YD, Abilash VJJoRI. Role of il-6 signalling in polycystic ovarian syndrome associated inflammation. 2020:103155.

[16] Peng Z, Sun Y, Lv X, Zhang H, Liu C, Dai SJPO. Interleukin-6 levels in women with polycystic ovary syndrome: a systematic review and meta-analysis. 2016;11(2):e0148531.

[17] Samy N, Hashim M, Sayed M, Said MJDm. *Clinical significance of inflammatory markers in polycystic ovary syndrome: their relationship to insulin resistance and body mass index.* 2009;26(4):163-70.

[18] Gao L, Gu Y, Yin XJPo. *High serum tumor necrosis factor-alpha levels in women with polycystic ovary syndrome: a meta-analysis.* 2016;11(10):e0164021.

[19] Stephens JM, Pekala PJJoBC. *Transcriptional repression of the GLUT4 and C/EBP genes in 3T3-L1 adipocytes by tumor necrosis factor-alpha.* 1991;266(32):21839-45.

[20] Amato G, Conte M, Mazziotti G, Lalli E, Vitolo G, Tucker AT, et al. *Serum and follicular fluid cytokines in polycystic ovary syndrome during stimulated cycles.* 2003;101(6):1177-82.

[21] Rostamtabar M, Esmaeilzadeh S, Tourani M, Rahmani A, Baee M, Shirafkan F, et al. *Pathophysiological roles of chronic low-grade inflammation mediators in polycystic ovary syndrome.* 2020;236(2):824-38.

[22] Yang Y, Qiao J, Li R, Li M-ZJRB, *Endocrinology. Is interleukin-18 associated with polycystic ovary syndrome?* 2011;9(1):7.

[23] Günther V, Alkatout I, Fuhs C, Salmassi A, Mettler L, Hedderich J, et al. *The Role of Interleukin-18 in Serum and Follicular Fluid during In Vitro Fertilization and Intracytoplasmic Sperm Injection.* 2016;2016.

[24] Matsumoto T, Kobayashi T, Kamata KJJoSMR. *Relationships among ET-1, PPARγ, oxidative stress and endothelial dysfunction in diabetic animals.* 2008;44(2):41-55.

[25] Koleva DI, Orbetzova MM, Nikolova JG, Tyutyundzhiev SBJAop, biochemistry. *Adipokines and soluble cell adhesion molecules in insulin resistant and non-insulin resistant women with polycystic ovary syndrome.* 2016;122(4):223-7.

[26] Solano ME, Sander VA, Ho H, Motta AB, Arck PCJJori. *Systemic inflammation, cellular influx and up-regulation of ovarian VCAM-1 expression in a mouse model of polycystic ovary syndrome (PCOS).* 2011;92(1-2):33-44.

[27] Candelaria NR, Padmanabhan A, Stossi F, Ljungberg MC, Shelly KE, Pew BK, et al. *VCAM1 is induced in ovarian theca and stromal cells in a mouse model of androgen excess.* 2019;160(6):1377-93.

[28] Holecki M, Zahorska-Markiewicz B, Janowska J, Nieszporek T, Wojaczynska-Stanek K, Zak-Golab A, et al. The influence of weight loss on serum osteoprotegerin concentration in obese perimenopausal women. *Obesity* (Silver Spring). 2007;15(8):1925-9.

[29] Ugur-Altun B, Altun A, Gerenli M, Tugrul A. The relationship between insulin resistance assessed by HOMA-IR and serum osteoprotegerin levels in obesity. *Diabetes Res Clin Pract.* 2005;68(3):217-22.

[30] Yang A, Pizzulli L, Luderitz B. Mean platelet volume as marker of restenosis after percutaneous transluminal coronary angioplasty in patients with stable and unstable angina pectoris. *Thromb Res.* 2006;117(4):371-7.

[31] Diamanti-Kandarakis E, Katsikis I, Piperi C, Kandaraki E, Piouka A, Papavassiliou AG, et al. Increased serum advanced glycation end-products is a distinct finding in lean women with polycystic ovary syndrome (PCOS). *Clin Endocrinol* (Oxf). 2008;69(4):634-41.

[32] Luque-Ramirez M, Alvarez-Blasco F, Botella-Carretero JI, Sanchon R, San Millan JL, Escobar-Morreale HF. Increased body iron stores of obese women with polycystic ovary syndrome are a consequence of insulin resistance and hyperinsulinism and are not a result of reduced menstrual losses. *Diabetes Care.* 2007;30(9):2309-13.

[33] Escobar-Morreale HF, Luque-Ramírez M, González F. Circulating inflammatory markers in polycystic ovary syndrome: a systematic review and metaanalysis. *Fertil Steril.* 2011;95(3):1048-58.e1-2.

[34] Lee H, Oh JY, Sung YA. Adipokines, insulin-like growth factor binding protein-3 levels, and insulin sensitivity in women with polycystic ovary syndrome. *Korean J Intern Med.* 2013;28(4):456-63.

[35] Keskin Kurt R, Okyay AG, Hakverdi AU, Gungoren A, Dolapcioglu KS, Karateke A, et al. The effect of obesity on inflammatory markers in patients with PCOS: a BMI-matched case-control study. *Arch Gynecol Obstet.* 2014;290(2):315-9.

[36] Donkena KV, Young CY, Tindall DJ. Oxidative stress and DNA methylation in prostate cancer. *Obstet Gynecol Int.* 2010;2010: 302051.

[37] Franco R, Schoneveld O, Georgakilas AG, Panayiotidis MI. Oxidative stress, DNA methylation and carcinogenesis. *Cancer Lett.* 2008;266(1):6-11.

[38] Touyz RM. Molecular and cellular mechanisms in vascular injury in hypertension: role of angiotensin II. *Curr Opin Nephrol Hypertens.* 2005;14(2):125-31.

[39] Siti HN, Kamisah Y, Kamsiah J. The role of oxidative stress, antioxidants and vascular inflammation in cardiovascular disease (a review). *Vascul Pharmacol.* 2015;71:40-56.

[40] Zuo T, Zhu M, Xu W. Roles of Oxidative Stress in Polycystic Ovary Syndrome and Cancers. *Oxid Med Cell Longev.* 2016;2016: 8589318.

[41] Alviggi C, Cariati F, Conforti A, De Rosa P, Vallone R, Strina I, et al. The effect of FT500 Plus((R)) on ovarian stimulation in PCOS women. *Reprod Toxicol.* 2016;59:40-4.

[42] de Groot PC, Dekkers OM, Romijn JA, Dieben SW, Helmerhorst FM. PCOS, coronary heart disease, stroke and the influence of obesity: a systematic review and meta-analysis. *Hum Reprod Update.* 2011;17(4):495-500.

[43] Nasiri N, Moini A, Eftekhari-Yazdi P, Karimian L, Salman-Yazdi R, Zolfaghari Z, et al. Abdominal obesity can induce both systemic and follicular fluid oxidative stress independent from polycystic ovary syndrome. *Eur J Obstet Gynecol Reprod Biol.* 2015;184:112-6.

[44] Murri M, Luque-Ramirez M, Insenser M, Ojeda-Ojeda M, Escobar-Morreale HF. Circulating markers of oxidative stress and polycystic ovary syndrome (PCOS): a systematic review and meta-analysis. *Hum Reprod Update.* 2013;19(3):268-88.

[45] Krstic J, Trivanovic D, Mojsilovic S, Santibanez JF. Transforming Growth Factor-Beta and Oxidative Stress Interplay: Implications in Tumorigenesis and Cancer Progression. *Oxid Med Cell Longev.* 2015;2015:654594.

[46] Reuter S, Gupta SC, Chaturvedi MM, Aggarwal BB. Oxidative stress, inflammation, and cancer: how are they linked? *Free Radic Biol Med.* 2010;49(11):1603-16.

[47] Dumesic DA, Lobo RA. Cancer risk and PCOS. *Steroids.* 2013;78(8):782-5.

[48] Khashchenko E, Vysokikh M, Uvarova E, Krechetova L, Vtorushina V, Ivanets T, et al. Activation of Systemic Inflammation and Oxidative Stress in Adolescent Girls with Polycystic Ovary Syndrome in Combination with Metabolic Disorders and Excessive Body Weight. *J Clin Med.* 2020;9(5).

[49] Melo ASd, Rodrigues JK, Junior AAJ, Ferriani RA, Navarro PA. Oxidative stress and polycystic ovary syndrome: an evaluation during ovarian stimulation for intracytoplasmic sperm injection. *J Reproduction.* 2017;153(1):97.

[50] March WA, Moore VM, Willson KJ, Phillips DI, Norman RJ, Davies MJ. The prevalence of polycystic ovary syndrome in a community sample assessed under contrasting diagnostic criteria. *Hum Reprod.* 2010;25(2):544-51.

[51] Giorgino F, Laviola L, Eriksson JW. Regional differences of insulin action in adipose tissue: insights from in vivo and in vitro studies. *Acta Physiol Scand.* 2005;183(1):13-30.

[52] Kirchengast S, Huber J. Body composition characteristics and body fat distribution in lean women with polycystic ovary syndrome. *Hum Reprod.* 2001;16(6):1255-60.

[53] Holguin F, Fitzpatrick A. Obesity, asthma, and oxidative stress. *J Appl Physiol* (1985). 2010;108(3):754-9.

[54] Choi HD, Kim JH, Chang MJ, Kyu-Youn Y, Shin WG. Effects of astaxanthin on oxidative stress in overweight and obese adults. *Phytother Res.* 2011;25(12):1813-8.

[55] Glintborg D. Endocrine and metabolic characteristics in polycystic ovary syndrome. *Dan Med J.* 2016;63(4).

[56] Tsouma I, Kouskouni E, Demeridou S, Boutsikou M, Hassiakos D, Chasiakou A, et al. Lipid lipoprotein profile alterations in Greek infertile women with polycystic ovaries: influence of adipocytokines levels. *In Vivo.* 2014;28(5):935-9.

[57] Ghaffarzad A, Amani R, Mehrzad Sadaghiani M, Darabi M, Cheraghian B. Correlation of Serum Lipoprotein Ratios with Insulin Resistance in Infertile Women with Polycystic Ovarian Syndrome: A Case Control Study. *Int J Fertil Steril.* 2016;10(1):29-35.

[58] Imran A, Butt MS, Arshad MS, Arshad MU, Saeed F, Sohaib M, et al. Exploring the potential of black tea based flavonoids against hyperlipidemia related disorders. *Lipids Health Dis.* 2018;17(1):57.

[59] Yang JT, Wang J, Zhou XR, Xiao C, Lou YY, Tang LH, et al. Luteolin alleviates cardiac ischemia/reperfusion injury in the hypercholesterolemic rat via activating Akt/Nrf2 signaling. *Naunyn Schmiedebergs Arch Pharmacol.* 2018;391(7):719-28.

[60] Ozata M, Mergen M, Oktenli C, Aydin A, Sanisoglu SY, Bolu E, et al. Increased oxidative stress and hypozincemia in male obesity. *Clin Biochem.* 2002;35(8):627-31.

[61] Furukawa S, Fujita T, Shimabukuro M, Iwaki M, Yamada Y, Nakajima Y, et al. Increased oxidative stress in obesity and its impact on metabolic syndrome. *J Clin Invest.* 2004;114(12):1752-61.

[62] Couillard C, Ruel G, Archer WR, Pomerleau S, Bergeron J, Couture P, et al. Circulating levels of oxidative stress markers and endothelial adhesion molecules in men with abdominal obesity. *J Clin Endocrinol Metab.* 2005;90(12):6454-9.

[63] Broughton DE, Moley KH. Obesity and female infertility: potential mediators of obesity's impact. *Fertil Steril.* 2017;107(4):840-7.

[64] Murri M, Luque-Ramírez M, Insenser M, Ojeda-Ojeda M, Escobar-Morreale HF. Circulating markers of oxidative stress and polycystic ovary syndrome (PCOS): a systematic review and meta-analysis. *Hum Reprod Update.* 2013;19(3):268-88.

[65] Zhang J, Fan P, Liu H, Bai H, Wang Y, Zhang F. Apolipoprotein A-I and B levels, dyslipidemia and metabolic syndrome in south-west Chinese women with PCOS. *Hum Reprod.* 2012;27(8):2484-93.

[66] Lim SS, Davies MJ, Norman RJ, Moran LJ. Overweight, obesity and central obesity in women with polycystic ovary syndrome: a systematic review and meta-analysis. *Hum Reprod Update.* 2012;18(6):618-37.

[67] Savic-Radojevic A, Bozic Antic I, Coric V, Bjekic-Macut J, Radic T, Zarkovic M, et al. Effect of hyperglycemia and hyperinsulinemia on glutathione peroxidase activity in non-obese women with polycystic ovary syndrome. *Hormones* (Athens). 2015;14(1):101-8.

[68] González F, Nair KS, Daniels JK, Basal E, Schimke JM. Hyperandrogenism sensitizes mononuclear cells to promote glucose-induced inflammation in lean reproductive-age women. *Am J Physiol Endocrinol Metab.* 2012;302(3):E297-306.

[69] Ciaraldi TP, Kolterman OG, Olefsky JM. Mechanism of the postreceptor defect in insulin action in human obesity. Decrease in glucose transport system activity. *J Clin Invest.* 1981;68(4):875-80.

[70] Klop B, Elte JW, Cabezas MC. Dyslipidemia in obesity: mechanisms and potential targets. *Nutrients.* 2013;5(4):1218-40.

[71] Yilmaz M, Biri A, Bukan N, Karakoç A, Sancak B, Törüner F, et al. Levels of lipoprotein and homocysteine in non-obese and obese patients with polycystic ovary syndrome. *Gynecol Endocrinol.* 2005;20(5):258-63.

[72] Salvadó L, Palomer X, Barroso E, Vázquez-Carrera M. Targeting endoplasmic reticulum stress in insulin resistance. *Trends Endocrinol Metab.* 2015;26(8):438-48.

[73] Mohamadin AM, Habib FA, Elahi TF. Serum paraoxonase 1 activity and oxidant/antioxidant status in Saudi women with polycystic ovary syndrome. *Pathophysiology.* 2010;17(3):189-96.

[74] Dias JP, Talbot S, Sénécal J, Carayon P, Couture R. Kinin B1 receptor enhances the oxidative stress in a rat model of insulin resistance: outcome in hypertension, allodynia and metabolic complications. *PLoS One.* 2010;5(9):e12622.

[75] Castro MC, Massa ML, Arbeláez LG, Schinella G, Gagliardino JJ, Francini F. Fructose-induced inflammation, insulin resistance and oxidative stress: A liver pathological triad effectively disrupted by lipoic acid. *Life Sci.* 2015;137:1-6.

[76] Rudich A, Kozlovsky N, Potashnik R, Bashan N. Oxidant stress reduces insulin responsiveness in 3T3-L1 adipocytes. *Am J Physiol.* 1997;272(5 Pt 1):E935-40.

[77] Evans JL, Maddux BA, Goldfine ID. The molecular basis for oxidative stress-induced insulin resistance. *Antioxid Redox Signal.* 2005;7(7-8):1040-52.

[78] González F. Inflammation in Polycystic Ovary Syndrome: underpinning of insulin resistance and ovarian dysfunction. *Steroids.* 2012;77(4):300-5.

[79] MacLaren R, Cui W, Simard S, Cianflone K. Influence of obesity and insulin sensitivity on insulin signaling genes in human omental and subcutaneous adipose tissue. *J Lipid Res.* 2008;49(2):308-23.

[80] Keane KN, Cruzat VF, Carlessi R, de Bittencourt PI, Jr., Newsholme P. Molecular Events Linking Oxidative Stress and Inflammation to Insulin Resistance and β-Cell Dysfunction. *Oxid Med Cell Longev.* 2015;2015:181643.

[81] Pollak M. The insulin and insulin-like growth factor receptor family in neoplasia: an update. *Nat Rev Cancer.* 2012;12(3):159-69.

[82] Barbieri RL, Makris A, Randall RW, Daniels G, Kistner RW, Ryan KJ. Insulin stimulates androgen accumulation in incubations of

ovarian stroma obtained from women with hyperandrogenism. *J Clin Endocrinol Metab.* 1986;62(5):904-10.

[83] Yelich JV, Wettemann RP, Marston TT, Spicer LJ. Luteinizing hormone, growth hormone, insulin-like growth factor-I, insulin and metabolites before puberty in heifers fed to gain at two rates. *Domest Anim Endocrinol.* 1996;13(4):325-38.

[84] González F. Inflammation in Polycystic Ovary Syndrome: underpinning of insulin resistance and ovarian dysfunction. *Steroids.* 2012;77(4):300-5.

[85] Nisenblat V, Norman RJ. Androgens and polycystic ovary syndrome. *Curr Opin Endocrinol Diabetes Obes.* 2009;16(3):224-31.

[86] González F, Minium J, Rote NS, Kirwan JP. Hyperglycemia alters tumor necrosis factor-alpha release from mononuclear cells in women with polycystic ovary syndrome. *J Clin Endocrinol Metab.* 2005;90(9):5336-42.

[87] Yang Y, Qiao J, Li R, Li MZ. Is interleukin-18 associated with polycystic ovary syndrome? *Reprod Biol Endocrinol.* 2011;9:7.

[88] Spaczynski RZ, Arici A, Duleba AJ. Tumor necrosis factor-alpha stimulates proliferation of rat ovarian theca-interstitial cells. *Biol Reprod.* 1999;61(4):993-8.

[89] González F, Nair KS, Daniels JK, Basal E, Schimke JM, Blair HE. Hyperandrogenism sensitizes leukocytes to hyperglycemia to promote oxidative stress in lean reproductive-age women. *J Clin Endocrinol Metab.* 2012;97(8):2836-43.

[90] Lu JP, Monardo L, Bryskin I, Hou ZF, Trachtenberg J, Wilson BC, et al. Androgens induce oxidative stress and radiation resistance in prostate cancer cells though NADPH oxidase. *Prostate Cancer Prostatic Dis.* 2010;13(1):39-46.

[91] González F, Rote NS, Minium J, Kirwan JP. Reactive oxygen species-induced oxidative stress in the development of insulin resistance and hyperandrogenism in polycystic ovary syndrome. *J Clin Endocrinol Metab.* 2006;91(1):336-40.

[92] Nikolić M, Macut D, Djordjevic A, Veličković N, Nestorović N, Bursać B, et al. Possible involvement of glucocorticoids in 5α-

dihydrotestosterone-induced PCOS-like metabolic disturbances in the rat visceral adipose tissue. *Mol Cell Endocrinol.* 2015;399:22-31.

[93] Tepavčević S, Milutinović DV, Macut D, Stanišić J, Nikolić M, Božić-Antić I, et al. Cardiac Nitric Oxide Synthases and Na^+/K^+-ATPase in the Rat Model of Polycystic Ovary Syndrome Induced by Dihydrotestosterone. *Exp Clin Endocrinol Diabetes.* 2015;123(5):303-7.

[94] Zheng YH, Ding T, Ye DF, Liu H, Lai MH, Ma HX. [Effect of low-frequency electroacupuncture intervention on oxidative stress and glucose metabolism in rats with polycystic ovary syndrome]. *Zhen Ci Yan Jiu.* 2015;40(2):125-30.

[95] Turan V, Sezer ED, Zeybek B, Sendag F. Infertility and the presence of insulin resistance are associated with increased oxidative stress in young, non-obese Turkish women with polycystic ovary syndrome. *J Pediatr Adolesc Gynecol.* 2015;28(2):119-23.

[96] Kurdoglu Z, Ozkol H, Tuluce Y, Koyuncu I. Oxidative status and its relation with insulin resistance in young non-obese women with polycystic ovary syndrome. *J Endocrinol Invest.* 2012;35(3):317-21.

[97] Ali HI, Elsadawy ME, Khater NH. Ultrasound assessment of polycystic ovaries: Ovarian volume and morphology; which is more accurate in making the diagnosis?! *The Egyptian Journal of Radiology and Nuclear Medicine.* 2016;47(1):347-50.

[98] Ikeda K, Baba T, Morishita M, Honnma H, Endo T, Kiya T, et al. Long-term treatment with dehydroepiandrosterone may lead to follicular atresia through interaction with anti-Mullerian hormone. *J Ovarian Res.* 2014;7:46.

[99] Lai Q, Xiang W, Li Q, Zhang H, Li Y, Zhu G, et al. Oxidative stress in granulosa cells contributes to poor oocyte quality and IVF-ET outcomes in women with polycystic ovary syndrome. *Front Med.* 2018;12(5):518-24.

[100] Adashi EY. Endocrinology of the ovary. *Hum Reprod.* 1994;9(5):815-27.

[101] Jakimiuk AJ, Weitsman SR, Navab A, Magoffin DA. Luteinizing hormone receptor, steroidogenesis acute regulatory protein, and

steroidogenic enzyme messenger ribonucleic acids are overexpressed in thecal and granulosa cells from polycystic ovaries. *J Clin Endocrinol Metab.* 2001;86(3):1318-23.

[102] Diamanti-Kandarakis E. Polycystic ovarian syndrome: pathophysiology, molecular aspects and clinical implications. *Expert Rev Mol Med.* 2008;10:e3.

[103] Pellatt L, Hanna L, Brincat M, Galea R, Brain H, Whitehead S, et al. Granulosa cell production of anti-Müllerian hormone is increased in polycystic ovaries. *J Clin Endocrinol Metab.* 2007;92(1):240-5.

[104] Xiong YL, Liang XY, Yang X, Li Y, Wei LN. Low-grade chronic inflammation in the peripheral blood and ovaries of women with polycystic ovarian syndrome. *Eur J Obstet Gynecol Reprod Biol.* 2011;159(1):148-50.

[105] Jancar N, Kopitar AN, Ihan A, Virant Klun I, Bokal EV. Effect of apoptosis and reactive oxygen species production in human granulosa cells on oocyte fertilization and blastocyst development. *J Assist Reprod Genet.* 2007;24(2-3):91-7.

[106] Wassarman PM, Litscher ES. Influence of the zona pellucida of the mouse egg on folliculogenesis and fertility. *Int J Dev Biol.* 2012;56(10-12):833-9.

[107] Balen AH, Tan SL, MacDougall J, Jacobs HS. Miscarriage rates following in-vitro fertilization are increased in women with polycystic ovaries and reduced by pituitary desensitization with buserelin. *Hum Reprod.* 1993;8(6):959-64.

[108] Morais R, Thomé R, Lemos F, Bazzoli N, Rizzo EJC, research t. Autophagy and apoptosis interplay during follicular atresia in fish ovary: a morphological and immunocytochemical study. 2012;347(2):467-78.

[109] González FJS. *Inflammation in polycystic ovary syndrome: underpinning of insulin resistance and ovarian dysfunction.* 2012;77(4):300-5.

[110] Xiong Yl, Liang XY, Yang X, Li Y, Wei LN. Low-grade chronic inflammation in the peripheral blood and ovaries of women with

polycystic ovarian syndrome. *European Journal of Obstetrics & Gynecology and Reproductive Biology.* 2011;159(1):148-50.

[111] Si Y, Zhao Y, Hao H, Liu J, Guo Y, Mu Y, et al. Infusion of mesenchymal stem cells ameliorates hyperglycemia in type 2 diabetic rats: identification of a novel role in improving insulin sensitivity. 2012;61(6):1616-25.

[112] Noorafshan A, Ahmadi M, Mesbah SF, Karbalay-Doust S. Stereological study of the effects of letrozole and estradiol valerate treatment on the ovary of rats. *Clin Exp Reprod Med.* 2013;40(3):115-21.

[113] Wood JR, Dumesic DA, Abbott DH, Strauss JF, 3rd. Molecular abnormalities in oocytes from women with polycystic ovary syndrome revealed by microarray analysis. *J Clin Endocrinol Metab.* 2007;92(2):705-13.

[114] Rice S, Ojha K, Whitehead S, Mason H. Stage-specific expression of androgen receptor, follicle-stimulating hormone receptor, and anti-Müllerian hormone type II receptor in single, isolated, human preantral follicles: relevance to polycystic ovaries. *J Clin Endocrinol Metab.* 2007;92(3):1034-40.

[115] Yang F, Ruan YC, Yang YJ, Wang K, Liang SS, Han YB, et al. Follicular hyperandrogenism downregulates aromatase in luteinized granulosa cells in polycystic ovary syndrome women. *Reproduction.* 2015;150(4):289-96.

[116] Balen AH. Hypersecretion of luteinizing hormone in the polycystic ovary syndrome and a novel hormone 'gonadotrophin surge attenuating factor'. *Journal of the Royal Society of Medicine.* 1995;88(6):339P-41P.

[117] Agarwal A, Aponte-Mellado A, Premkumar BJ, Shaman A, Gupta S. The effects of oxidative stress on female reproduction: a review. *Reproductive Biology and Endocrinology.* 2012;10(1):49.

[118] Devine PJ, Perreault SD, Luderer U. Roles of reactive oxygen species and antioxidants in ovarian toxicity. *Biol Reprod.* 2012;86(2):27.

[119] Becatti M, Fucci R, Mannucci A, Barygina V, Mugnaini M, Criscuoli L, et al. A Biochemical Approach to Detect Oxidative Stress in

Infertile Women Undergoing Assisted Reproductive Technology Procedures. *Int J Mol Sci.* 2018;19(2).
[120] Nishihara T, Matsumoto K, Hosoi Y, Morimoto YJRm, biology. *Evaluation of antioxidant status and oxidative stress markers in follicular fluid for human in vitro fertilization outcome.* 2018;17(4):481-6.
[121] Fabjan T, Bokal EV, Klun IV, Bedenk J, Kumer K, Osredkar J. Antimüllerian Hormone and Oxidative Stress Biomarkers as Predictors of Successful Preg-nancy in Polycystic Ovary Syndrome, Endometriosis and Tubal Infertility Factor. 2020. 2020;67(3):11. *J Acta Chimica Slovenica.*
[122] Liu Y, Yu Z, Zhao S, Cheng L, Man Y, Gao X, et al. Oxidative stress markers in the follicular fluid of patients with polycystic ovary syndrome correlate with a decrease in embryo quality. *J Assist Reprod Genet.* 2020.
[123] Morais RDVS, Thomé RG, Lemos FS, Bazzoli N, Rizzo E. Autophagy and apoptosis interplay during follicular atresia in fish ovary: a morphological and immunocytochemical study. *Cell and Tissue Research.* 2012;347(2):467-78.
[124] Nakahara K, Saito H, Saito T, Ito M, Ohta N, Takahashi T, et al. The incidence of apoptotic bodies in membrana granulosa can predict prognosis of ova from patients participating in in vitro fertilization programs. *Fertil Steril.* 1997;68(2):312-7.
[125] Seino T, Saito H, Kaneko T, Takahashi T, Kawachiya S, Kurachi H. Eight-hydroxy-2'-deoxyguanosine in granulosa cells is correlated with the quality of oocytes and embryos in an in vitro fertilization-embryo transfer program. *Fertil Steril.* 2002;77(6):1184-90.
[126] Banaszewska B, Pawelczyk L, Spaczynski R. Current and future aspects of several adjunctive treatment strategies in polycystic ovary syndrome. *Reproductive biology.* 2019;19(4):309-15.
[127] Artini PG, Obino MER, Sergiampietri C, Pinelli S, Papini F, Casarosa E, et al. PCOS and pregnancy: a review of available therapies to improve the outcome of pregnancy in women with polycystic ovary

syndrome. *Expert review of endocrinology & metabolism.* 2018;13(2):87-98.

[128] Smits RM, Mackenzie-Proctor R, Fleischer K, Showell MG. Antioxidants in fertility: Impact on male and female reproductive outcomes. *Fertility and Sterility.* 2018;110(4):578-80.

[129] Agarwal A, Durairajanayagam D, Du Plessis SS. Utility of antioxidants during assisted reproductive techniques: an evidence based review. *Reproductive Biology and Endocrinology.* 2014;12(1):112.

[130] Showell MG, Mackenzie-Proctor R, Jordan V, Hart RJ. Antioxidants for female subfertility. *Cochrane Database of Systematic Reviews.* 2020(8).

[131] Showell MG, Mackenzie-Proctor R, Jordan V, Hodgson R, Farquhar C. Inositol for subfertile women with polycystic ovary syndrome. *Cochrane Database of Systematic Reviews.* 2018(12).

[132] Artini PG, Di Berardino O, Papini F, Genazzani A, Simi G, Ruggiero M, et al. Endocrine and clinical effects of myo-inositol administration in polycystic ovary syndrome. A randomized study. *Gynecological Endocrinology.* 2013;29(4):375-9.

[133] Bevilacqua A, Bizzarri M. Physiological role and clinical utility of inositols in polycystic ovary syndrome. *Best Practice & Research Clinical Obstetrics & Gynaecology.* 2016;37:129-39.

[134] Lisi F. Pretreatment with myo-inositol in patients undergoing gonadotropins multiple follicular stimulation for IVF. *Acta Medica International.* 2016;3(1):8.

[135] Papaleo E, Molgora M, Quaranta L, Pellegrino M, De Michele F. Myo-inositol products in polycystic ovary syndrome (PCOS) treatment: quality, labeling accuracy, and cost comparison. *Eur Rev Med Pharmacol Sci.* 2011;15(2):165-74.

[136] Pundir J, Psaroudakis D, Savnur P, Bhide P, Sabatini L, Teede H, et al. Inositol treatment of anovulation in women with polycystic ovary syndrome: a meta-analysis of randomised trials. BJOG: An *International Journal of Obstetrics & Gynaecology.* 2018;125(3): 299-308.

[137] Januszewski M, Issat T, Jakimiuk AA, Santor-Zaczynska M, Jakimiuk AJ. Metabolic and hormonal effects of a combined Myo-inositol and d-chiro-inositol therapy on patients with polycystic ovary syndrome (PCOS). *Ginekologia polska.* 2019;90(1):7-10.

[138] Maleki V, Jafari-Vayghan H, Kashani A, Moradi F, Vajdi M, Kheirouri S, et al. Potential roles of carnitine in patients with polycystic ovary syndrome: a systematic review. *Gynecological Endocrinology.* 2019;35(6):463-9.

[139] Laganà AS, Garzon S, Casarin J, Franchi M, Ghezzi F. Inositol in polycystic ovary syndrome: restoring fertility through a pathophysiology-based approach. *Trends in endocrinology & metabolism.* 2018;29(11):768-80.

[140] Sene AA, Tabatabaie A, Nikniaz H, Alizadeh A, Sheibani K, Alisaraie MM, et al. The myo-inositol effect on the oocyte quality and fertilization rate among women with polycystic ovary syndrome undergoing assisted reproductive technology cycles: a randomized clinical trial. *Archives of gynecology and obstetrics.* 2019; 299(6):1701-7.

[141] Kitano Y, Hashimoto S, Matsumoto H, Yamochi T, Yamanaka M, Nakaoka Y, et al. Oral administration of l-carnitine improves the clinical outcome of fertility in patients with IVF treatment. *Gynecological Endocrinology.* 2018;34(8):684-8.

[142] Mojaverrostami S, Asghari N, Khamisabadi M, Khoei HH. The role of melatonin in polycystic ovary syndrome: a review. *International Journal of Reproductive BioMedicine.* 2019;17(12):865.

[143] Jain P, Jain M, Haldar C, Singh TB, Jain S. Melatonin and its correlation with testosterone in polycystic ovarian syndrome. *Journal of human reproductive sciences.* 2013;6(4):253.

[144] Hasan KN, Maitra SK. *Melatonin in the Clinical Management of Polycystic Ovarian Syndrome.*

[145] Woo MM, Tai CJ, Kang SK, Nathwani PS, Pang SF, Leung PC. Direct action of melatonin in human granulosa-luteal cells. *The Journal of Clinical Endocrinology & Metabolism.* 2001;86 (10):4789-97.

[146] Tamura H, Nakamura Y, Korkmaz A, Manchester LC, Tan DX, Sugino N, et al. Melatonin and the ovary: physiological and pathophysiological implications. *Fertility and Sterility.* 2009;92(1): 328-43.

[147] Tamura H, Takasaki A, Miwa I, Taniguchi K, Maekawa R, Asada H, et al. Oxidative stress impairs oocyte quality and melatonin protects oocytes from free radical damage and improves fertilization rate. *Journal of pineal research.* 2008;44(3):280-7.

[148] Eryilmaz OG, Devran A, Sarikaya E, Aksakal FN, Mollamahmutoğlu L, Cicek N. Melatonin improves the oocyte and the embryo in IVF patients with sleep disturbances, but does not improve the sleeping problems. *Journal of Assisted Reproduction and Genetics.* 2011;28(9):815.

[149] Batıoğlu AS, Şahin U, Gürlek B, Öztürk N, Ünsal E. The efficacy of melatonin administration on oocyte quality. *Gynecological Endocrinology.* 2012;28(2):91-3.

[150] Tagliaferri V, Romualdi D, Scarinci E, Cicco SD, Florio CD, Immediata V, et al. Melatonin treatment may be able to restore menstrual cyclicity in women with PCOS: a pilot study. *Reproductive Sciences.* 2018;25(2):269-75.

[151] Pacchiarotti A, Carlomagno G, Antonini G, Pacchiarotti A. Effect of myo-inositol and melatonin versus myo-inositol, in a randomized controlled trial, for improving in vitro fertilization of patients with polycystic ovarian syndrome. *Gynecological Endocrinology.* 2016;32(1):69-73.

[152] Seko LM, Moroni RM, Leitao VM, Teixeira DM, Nastri CO, Martins WP. Melatonin supplementation during controlled ovarian stimulation for women undergoing assisted reproductive technology: systematic review and meta-analysis of randomized controlled trials. *Fertility and Sterility.* 2014;101(1):154-61. e4.

[153] Javanmanesh F, Kashanian M, Rahimi M, Sheikhansari N. A comparison between the effects of metformin and N-acetyl cysteine (NAC) on some metabolic and endocrine characteristics of women

with polycystic ovary syndrome. *Gynecological Endocrinology.* 2016;32(4):285-9.

[154] Sacchinelli A, Venturella R, Lico D, Di Cello A, Lucia A, Rania E, et al. The efficacy of inositol and N-acetyl cysteine administration (Ovaric HP) in improving the ovarian function in infertile women with PCOS with or without insulin resistance. *Obstetrics and gynecology international.* 2014;2014.

[155] Oner G, Muderris II. Clinical, endocrine and metabolic effects of metformin vs N-acetyl-cysteine in women with polycystic ovary syndrome. *European Journal of Obstetrics & Gynecology and Reproductive Biology.* 2011;159(1):127-31.

[156] Della Corte L, Foreste V, Barra F, Gustavino C, Alessandri F, Centurioni MG, et al. Current and experimental drug therapy for the treatment of polycystic ovarian syndrome. *Expert Opinion on Investigational Drugs.* 2020;29(8):819-30.

[157] Saha L, Kaur S, Saha PK. N-acetyl cysteine in clomiphene citrate resistant polycystic ovary syndrome: A review of reported outcomes. *Journal of pharmacology & pharmacotherapeutics.* 2013;4(3):187.

[158] Mostajeran F, Tehrani HG, Rahbary B. N-Acetylcysteine as an Adjuvant to Letrozole for Induction of Ovulation in Infertile Patients with Polycystic Ovary Syndrome. *Advanced biomedical research.* 2018;7.

[159] Devi N, Boya C, Chhabra M, Bansal D. N-acetyl-cysteine as adjuvant therapy in female infertility: a systematic review and meta-analysis. *Journal of Basic and Clinical Physiology and Pharmacology.* 2020;1(ahead-of-print).

[160] Thakker D, Raval A, Patel I, Walia R. N-acetylcysteine for polycystic ovary syndrome: a systematic review and meta-analysis of randomized controlled clinical trials. *Obstetrics and gynecology international.* 2015;2015.

[161] Elgindy EA, El-Huseiny AM, Mostafa MI, Gaballah AM, Ahmed TA. N-acetyl cysteine: could it be an effective adjuvant therapy in ICSI cycles? A preliminary study. *Reproductive biomedicine online.* 2010;20(6):789-96.

[162] Cheraghi E, Mehranjani MS, Shariatzadeh MA, Esfahani MHN, Ebrahimi Z. N-Acetylcysteine improves oocyte and embryo quality in polycystic ovary syndrome patients undergoing intracytoplasmic sperm injection: an alternative to metformin. *Reproduction, Fertility and Development.* 2016;28(6):723-31.

[163] Vanella A, Russo A, Acquaviva R, Campisi A, Di Giacomo C, Sorrenti V, et al. L-propionyl-carnitine as superoxide scavenger, antioxidant, and DNA cleavage protector. *Cell Biology and Toxicology.* 2000;16(2):99-104.

[164] Abdelrazik H, Agrawal A. L-carnitine and assisted reproduction. *Arch Med Sci.* 2009;5:43-7.

[165] Agarwal A, Sengupta P, Durairajanayagam D. Role of L-carnitine in female infertility. *Reproductive Biology and Endocrinology.* 2018;16(1):5.

[166] Surai PF. Antioxidant action of carnitine: molecular mechanisms and practical applications. *EC Veterinary Science.* 2015;2(1):66-84.

[167] Jamilian H, Jamilian M, Samimi M, Afshar Ebrahimi F, Rahimi M, Bahmani F, et al. Oral carnitine supplementation influences mental health parameters and biomarkers of oxidative stress in women with polycystic ovary syndrome: a randomized, double-blind, placebo-controlled trial. *Gynecological Endocrinology.* 2017;33(6):442-7.

[168] Samimi M, Jamilian M, Ebrahimi FA, Rahimi M, Tajbakhsh B, Asemi Z. Oral carnitine supplementation reduces body weight and insulin resistance in women with polycystic ovary syndrome: a randomized, double-blind, placebo-controlled trial. *Clinical endocrinology.* 2016;84(6):851-7.

[169] Fathizadeh H, Milajerdi A, Reiner Ž, Amirani E, Asemi Z, Mansournia MA, et al. The effects of L-carnitine supplementation on indicators of inflammation and oxidative stress: a systematic review and meta-analysis of randomized controlled trials. *Journal of Diabetes & Metabolic Disorders.* 2020:1-16.

[170] Ismail AM, Hamed AH, Saso S, Thabet HH. Adding L-carnitine to clomiphene resistant PCOS women improves the quality of ovulation and the pregnancy rate. A randomized clinical trial. *European Journal*

of *Obstetrics & Gynecology and Reproductive Biology.* 2014;180:148-52.

[171] Florou P, Anagnostis P, Theocharis P, Chourdakis M, Goulis DG. Does coenzyme Q 10 supplementation improve fertility outcomes in women undergoing assisted reproductive technology procedures? A systematic review and meta-analysis of randomized-controlled trials. *Journal of Assisted Reproduction and Genetics.* 2020:1-11.

[172] Paul M, Baker M, Williams RN, Bowrey DJ. Nutritional support and dietary interventions following esophagectomy: challenges and solutions. *Nutrition and Dietary Supplements.* 2017;9:9-21.

[173] Bentov Y, Hannam T, Jurisicova A, Esfandiari N, Casper RF. Coenzyme Q10 supplementation and oocyte aneuploidy in women undergoing IVF-ICSI treatment. *Clinical Medicine Insights: Reproductive Health.* 2014;8:CMRH. S14681.

[174] Xu Y, Nisenblat V, Lu C, Li R, Qiao J, Zhen X, et al. Pretreatment with coenzyme Q10 improves ovarian response and embryo quality in low-prognosis young women with decreased ovarian reserve: a randomized controlled trial. *Reproductive Biology and Endocrinology.* 2018;16(1):29.

[175] Caballero T, Fiameni F, Valcarcel A, Buzzi J. Dietary supplementation with coenzyme Q10 in poor responder patients undergoing IVF-ICSI Treatment. *Fertility and Sterility.* 2016;106(3):e58.

[176] El Refaeey A, Selem A, Badawy A. Combined coenzyme Q10 and clomiphene citrate for ovulation induction in clomiphene-citrate-resistant polycystic ovary syndrome. *Reproductive biomedicine online.* 2014;29(1):119-24.

[177] Sen Sharma S, editor Co-enzyme Q10-A mitochondrial antioxidant a new hope for success in infertility in clomiphene-citrate-resistant polycystic ovary syndrome. *BJOG-AN International Journal of Obstetrics and Gynaecology;* 2017: Wiley 111 River St, Hoboken 07030-5774, NJ USA.

[178] Liu M, Zhu H, Hu X, Zhu Y, Chen H. Efficacy of coenzyme Q10 supplementation on glucose metabolism, lipid profiles, and

biomarkers of inflammation in women with polycystic ovary syndrome: A protocol for a systematic review and meta-analysis. *Medicine*. 2020;99(46).

[179] Samimi M, Zarezade Mehrizi M, Foroozanfard F, Akbari H, Jamilian M, Ahmadi S, et al. The effects of coenzyme Q10 supplementation on glucose metabolism and lipid profiles in women with polycystic ovary syndrome: a randomized, double-blind, placebo-controlled trial. *Clinical endocrinology*. 2017;86(4):560-6.

[180] Yahya AA, Abdulridha MK, Al-Rubuyae BJ, Al-Atar HA. The Effect of Vitamin D and Co-enzyme Q10 Replacement Therapy on Hormonal Profile and Ovulation Statusin Women with Clomiphene Citrate Resistant Polycystic Ovary Syndrome. *Journal of Pharmaceutical Sciences and Research*. 2019;11(1):208-15.

[181] Al-Qadhi HI, Kadhim EJ, Ali RH. Coenzyme Q10 effects on body weight, serum testosterone level and oxidative stress in women with polycystic ovarian syndrome (PCOS). *International Journal of Research in Pharmaceutical Sciences*. 2017;8(3):377-82.

[182] Izadi A, Ebrahimi S, Shirazi S, Taghizadeh S, Parizad M, Farzadi L, et al. Hormonal and metabolic effects of coenzyme Q10 and/or vitamin E in patients with polycystic ovary syndrome. *The Journal of Clinical Endocrinology & Metabolism*. 2019;104(2):319-27.

[183] Geva E, Bartoov B, Zabludovsky N, Lessing JB, Lerner-Geva L, Amit A. The effect of antioxidant treatment on human spermatozoa and fertilization rate in an in vitro fertilization program. *Fertility and Sterility*. 1996;66(3):430-4.

[184] Ghanem H, Shaeer O, El-Segini A. Combination clomiphene citrate and antioxidant therapy for idiopathic male infertility: a randomized controlled trial. *Fertility and Sterility*. 2010;93(7):2232-5.

[185] Saleh H, Omar E, Froemming G, Said R. Tocotrienol preserves ovarian function in cyclophosphamide therapy. *Human & experimental toxicology*. 2015;34(10):946-52.

[186] Riley JC, Behrman HR. Oxygen radicals and reactive oxygen species in reproduction. *Proceedings of the Society for Experimental Biology and Medicine*. 1991;198(3):781-91.

[187] Morsy AA, Sabri NA, Mourad AM, Mojahed EM, Shawki MA. Randomized controlled open-label study of the effect of vitamin E supplementation on fertility in clomiphene citrate-resistant polycystic ovary syndrome. *Journal of Obstetrics and Gynaecology Research.* 2020;46(11):2375-82.

[188] Fatemi F, Mohammadzadeh A, Sadeghi MR, Akhondi MM, Mohammadmoradi S, Kamali K, et al. Role of vitamin E and D3 supplementation in Intra-Cytoplasmic Sperm Injection outcomes of women with polycystic ovarian syndrome: A double blinded randomized placebo-controlled trial. *Clinical nutrition ESPEN.* 2017;18:23-30.

[189] Cicek N, Eryilmaz OG, Sarikaya E, Gulerman C, Genc Y. Vitamin E effect on controlled ovarian stimulation of unexplained infertile women. *Journal of Assisted Reproduction and Genetics.* 2012;29(4):325-8.

[190] Mohammadi M. Oxidative stress and polycystic ovary syndrome: a brief review. *International journal of preventive medicine.* 2019;10.

[191] Griesinger G, Franke K, Kinast C, Kutzelnigg A, Riedinger S, Kulin S, et al. Ascorbic acid supplement during luteal phase in IVF. *Journal of Assisted Reproduction and Genetics.* 2002;19(4):164-8.

[192] Henmi H, Endo T, Kitajima Y, Manase K, Hata H, Kudo R. Effects of ascorbic acid supplementation on serum progesterone levels in patients with a luteal phase defect. *Fertility and Sterility.* 2003;80(2):459-61.

[193] Panti AA, Shehu CE, Saidu Y, Tunau KA, Nwobodo EI, Jimoh A, et al. Oxidative stress and outcome of antioxidant supplementation in patients with polycystic ovarian syndrome (PCOS). *Int J Reprod Contracept Obstet Gynecol.* 2018;7:1667-72.

[194] Christakos S, Ajibade DV, Dhawan P, Fechner AJ, Mady LJ. Vitamin D: metabolism. *Rheumatic Disease Clinics.* 2012;38(1):1-11.

[195] Ramagopalan SV, Heger A, Berlanga AJ, Maugeri NJ, Lincoln MR, Burrell A, et al. A ChIP-seq defined genome-wide map of vitamin D receptor binding: associations with disease and evolution. *Genome research.* 2010;20(10):1352-60.

[196] He C, Lin Z, Robb SW, Ezeamama AE. Serum vitamin D levels and polycystic ovary syndrome: a systematic review and meta-analysis. *Nutrients.* 2015;7(6):4555-77.

[197] Teegarden D, Donkin SS. Vitamin D: emerging new roles in insulin sensitivity. *Nutrition research reviews.* 2009;22(1):82-92.

[198] De Groot PC, Dekkers OM, Romijn JA, Dieben SW, Helmerhorst FM. PCOS, coronary heart disease, stroke and the influence of obesity: a systematic review and meta-analysis. *Human reproduction update.* 2011;17(4):495-500.

[199] Verdoia M, Schaffer A, Sartori C, Barbieri L, Cassetti E, Marino P, et al. Vitamin D deficiency is independently associated with the extent of coronary artery disease. *European journal of clinical investigation.* 2014;44(7):634-42.

[200] Song Y, Wang L, Pittas AG, Del Gobbo LC, Zhang C, Manson JE, et al. Blood 25-hydroxy vitamin D levels and incident type 2 diabetes: a meta-analysis of prospective studies. *Am Diabetes Assoc;* 2013.

[201] Khan H, Kunutsor S, Franco OH, Chowdhury R. Vitamin D, type 2 diabetes and other metabolic outcomes: a systematic review and meta-analysis of prospective studies. *Proceedings of the Nutrition Society.* 2013;72(1):89-97.

[202] Chu J, Gallos I, Tobias A, Tan B, Eapen A, Coomarasamy A. Vitamin D and assisted reproductive treatment outcome: a systematic review and meta-analysis. *Human reproduction.* 2018;33(1):65-80.

[203] Zhao J, Huang X, Xu B, Yan Y, Zhang Q, Li Y. Whether vitamin D was associated with clinical outcome after IVF/ICSI: a systematic review and meta-analysis. *Reproductive Biology and Endocrinology.* 2018;16(1):1-7.

[204] Cozzolino M, Busnelli A, Pellegrini L, Riviello E, Vitagliano A. How vitamin D level influences in vitro fertilization outcomes: results of a systematic review and meta-analysis. *Fertility and Sterility.* 2020.

[205] Paffoni A, Somigliana E, Sarais V, Ferrari S, Reschini M, Makieva S, et al. Effect of vitamin D supplementation on assisted reproduction technology (ART) outcomes and underlying biological mechanisms: protocol of a randomized clinical controlled trial. The

"supplementation of vitamin D and reproductive outcome"(SUNDRO) study. *BMC pregnancy and childbirth.* 2019;19(1):1-9.

[206] Omran EF, Ramzy A, Shohayeb A, Farouk N, Soliman M, Baz H, et al. Relation of serum vitamin D level in polycystic ovarian syndrome (PCOS) patients to ICSI outcome. *Middle East Fertility Society Journal.* 2020;25(1):1-8.

[207] Dastorani M, Aghadavod E, Mirhosseini N, Foroozanfard F, Modarres SZ, Siavashani MA, et al. The effects of vitamin D supplementation on metabolic profiles and gene expression of insulin and lipid metabolism in infertile polycystic ovary syndrome candidates for in vitro fertilization. *Reproductive Biology and Endocrinology.* 2018;16(1):1-7.

[208] Qazi IH, Angel C, Yang H, Pan B, Zoidis E, Zeng CJ, et al. Selenium, selenoproteins, and female reproduction: a review. *Molecules.* 2018;23(12):3053.

[209] Zoidis E, Seremelis I, Kontopoulos N, Danezis GP. Selenium-dependent antioxidant enzymes: Actions and properties of selenoproteins. *Antioxidants.* 2018;7(5):66.

[210] Papp LV, Lu J, Holmgren A, Khanna KK. From selenium to selenoproteins: synthesis, identity, and their role in human health. *Antioxidants & redox signaling.* 2007;9(7):775-806.

[211] Luddi A, Capaldo A, Focarelli R, Gori M, Morgante G, Piomboni P, et al. Antioxidants reduce oxidative stress in follicular fluid of aged women undergoing IVF. *Reproductive Biology and Endocrinology.* 2016;14(1):1-7.

[212] Jiménez Tuñón JM, Trilles PP, Molina MG, Duvison MH, Pastor BM, Martín PS, et al. A Double-blind, randomized prospective study to evaluate the efficacy of previous therapy with melatonin, myo-inositol, folic acid, and selenium in improving the results of an assisted reproductive treatment. *Clinical Medicine Insights: Therapeutics.* 2017;9:1179559X17742902.

[213] Atef MM, Abd-Ellatif RN, Emam MN, Amer AI, Hafez YM. Therapeutic potential of sodium selenite in letrozole induced

polycystic ovary syndrome rat model: Targeting mitochondrial approach (selenium in PCOS). *Archives of biochemistry and biophysics*. 2019;671:245-54.

[214] Heidar Z, Hamzepour N, Modarres SZ, Mirzamoradi M, Aghadavod E, Pourhanifeh MH, et al. The effects of selenium supplementation on clinical symptoms and gene expression related to inflammation and vascular endothelial growth factor in infertile women candidate for in vitro fertilization. *Biological trace element research*. 2020;193(2):319-25.

[215] Jamilian M, Mansury S, Bahmani F, Heidar Z, Amirani E, Asemi Z. The effects of probiotic and selenium co-supplementation on parameters of mental health, hormonal profiles, and biomarkers of inflammation and oxidative stress in women with polycystic ovary syndrome. *Journal of ovarian research*. 2018;11(1):1-7.

[216] Köse SA, Nazıroğlu M. Selenium reduces oxidative stress and calcium entry through TRPV1 channels in the neutrophils of patients with polycystic ovary syndrome. *Biological trace element research*. 2014;158(2):136-42.

[217] Mintziori G, Mousiolis A, Duntas LH, Goulis DG. Evidence for a manifold role of selenium in infertility. *Hormones*. 2020;19(1):55-9.

[218] Wang Z, Zhai D, Zhang D, Bai L, Yao R, Yu J, et al. Quercetin decreases insulin resistance in a polycystic ovary syndrome rat model by improving inflammatory microenvironment. *Reproductive Sciences*. 2017;24(5):682-90.

[219] Lakhanpal P, Rai DK. Quercetin: a versatile flavonoid. *Internet Journal of Medical Update*. 2007;2(2):22-37.

[220] Boots AW, Haenen GR, Bast A. Health effects of quercetin: from antioxidant to nutraceutical. *European journal of pharmacology*. 2008;585(2-3):325-37.

[221] Lesjak M, Beara I, Simin N, Pintać D, Majkić T, Bekvalac K, et al. Antioxidant and anti-inflammatory activities of quercetin and its derivatives. *Journal of Functional Foods*. 2018;40:68-75.

[222] Li Y, Yao J, Han C, Yang J, Chaudhry MT, Wang S, et al. Quercetin, inflammation and immunity. *Nutrients*. 2016;8(3):167.

[223] Faggio C, Sureda A, Morabito S, Sanches-Silva A, Mocan A, Nabavi SF, et al. Flavonoids and platelet aggregation: a brief review. *European journal of pharmacology*. 2017;807:91-101.
[224] Shen Y, Croft KD, Hodgson JM, Kyle R, Lee ILE, Wang Y, et al. Quercetin and its metabolites improve vessel function by inducing eNOS activity via phosphorylation of AMPK. *Biochemical pharmacology*. 2012;84(8):1036-44.
[225] Bondonno NP, Bondonno CP, Hodgson JM, Ward NC, Croft KD. The efficacy of quercetin in cardiovascular health. *Current Nutrition Reports*. 2015;4(4):290-303.
[226] Perez-Vizcaino F, Duarte J, Jimenez R, Santos-Buelga C, Osuna A. Antihypertensive effects of the flavonoid quercetin. *Pharmacological Reports*. 2009;61(1):67-75.
[227] Shi GJ, Li Y, Cao QH, Wu HX, Tang XY, Gao XH, et al. In vitro and in vivo evidence that quercetin protects against diabetes and its complications: A systematic review of the literature. *Biomedicine & Pharmacotherapy*. 2019;109:1085-99.
[228] M Eid H, S Haddad P. The antidiabetic potential of quercetin: underlying mechanisms. *Current medicinal chemistry*. 2017;24(4):355-64.
[229] Gurav M, Bhise S, Warghade S. Effect of Quercetin on Beta cell regeneration. *Asian J Pharm Pharmacol*. 2018;4:214-21.
[230] Bentz AB. A review of Quercetin: chemistry, Antioxident properties, and bioavailability. *Journal of young investigators*. 2017.
[231] Tabrizi FPF, Hajizadeh-Sharafabad F, Vaezi M, Jafari-Vayghan H, Alizadeh M, Maleki V. Quercetin and polycystic ovary syndrome, current evidence and future directions: a systematic review. *Journal of ovarian research*. 2020;13(1):11.
[232] Jahan S, Abid A, Khalid S, Afsar T, Shaheen G, Almajwal A, et al. Therapeutic potentials of Quercetin in management of polycystic ovarian syndrome using Letrozole induced rat model: a histological and a biochemical study. *Journal of ovarian research*. 2018;11(1):1-10.

[233] Neisy A, Zal F, Seghatoleslam A, Alaee S. Amelioration by quercetin of insulin resistance and uterine GLUT4 and ERα gene expression in rats with polycystic ovary syndrome (PCOS). *Reproduction, Fertility and Development.* 2019;31(2):315-23.

[234] Shah KN, Patel SS. Phosphatidylinositide 3-kinase inhibition: A new potential target for the treatment of polycystic ovarian syndrome. *Pharmaceutical biology.* 2016;54(6):975-83.

[235] Hong Y, Yin Y, Tan Y, Hong K, Jiang F, Wang Y. Effect of quercetin on biochemical parameters in letrozoleinduced polycystic ovary syndrome in rats. *Tropical Journal of Pharmaceutical Research.* 2018;17(9):1783-8.

[236] Rezvan N, Moini A, Janani L, Mohammad K, Saedisomeolia A, Nourbakhsh M, et al. Effects of quercetin on adiponectin-mediated insulin sensitivity in polycystic ovary syndrome: a randomized placebo-controlled double-blind clinical trial. *Hormone and Metabolic Research.* 2017;49(02):115-21.

[237] Khorshidi M, Moini A, Alipoor E, Rezvan N, Gorgani-Firuzjaee S, Yaseri M, et al. The effects of quercetin supplementation on metabolic and hormonal parameters as well as plasma concentration and gene expression of resistin in overweight or obese women with polycystic ovary syndrome. *Phytotherapy research.* 2018;32(11):2282-9.

[238] Rezvan N, Moini A, Gorgani-Firuzjaee S, Hosseinzadeh-Attar MJ. Oral quercetin supplementation enhances adiponectin receptor transcript expression in polycystic ovary syndrome patients: a randomized placebo-controlled double-blind clinical trial. *Cell Journal* (Yakhteh). 2018;19(4):627.

[239] Wang L, Qi H, Baker PN, Zhen Q, Zeng Q, Shi R, et al. Altered Circulating Inflammatory Cytokines Are Associated with Anovulatory Polycystic Ovary Syndrome (PCOS) Women Resistant to Clomiphene Citrate Treatment. *Med Sci Monit.* 2017;23:1083-9.

[240] Hasanpour Dehkordi A, Abbaszadeh A, Mir S, Hasanvand A. Metformin and its anti-inflammatory and anti-oxidative effects; new concepts. *Journal of Renal Injury Prevention.* 2019.

[241] An H, He L. Current understanding of metformin effect on the control of hyperglycemia in diabetes. *The Journal of endocrinology.* 2016;228(3):R97.

[242] Mansfield R, Galea R, Brincat M, Hole D, Mason H. Metformin has direct effects on human ovarian steroidogenesis. *Fertility and Sterility.* 2003;79(4):956-62.

[243] Teede HJ, Misso ML, Costello MF, Dokras A, Laven J, Moran L, et al. Recommendations from the international evidence-based guideline for the assessment and management of polycystic ovary syndrome. *Human reproduction.* 2018;33(9):1602-18.

[244] Morley LC, Tang T, Yasmin E, Norman RJ, Balen AH. Insulin-sensitising drugs (metformin, rosiglitazone, pioglitazone, D-chiro-inositol) for women with polycystic ovary syndrome, oligo amenorrhoea and subfertility. *Cochrane Database of Systematic Reviews.* 2017(11).

[245] Bordewijk EM, Nahuis M, Costello MF, Van der Veen F, Tso LO, Mol BWJ, et al. Metformin during ovulation induction with gonadotrophins followed by timed intercourse or intrauterine insemination for subfertility associated with polycystic ovary syndrome. *Cochrane Database of Systematic Reviews.* 2017(1).

[246] Kjøtrød S, Carlsen S, Rasmussen P, Holst-Larsen T, Mellembakken J, Thurin-Kjellberg A, et al. Use of metformin before and during assisted reproductive technology in non-obese young infertile women with polycystic ovary syndrome: a prospective, randomized, double-blind, multi-centre study. *Human reproduction.* 2011;26(8):2045-53.

[247] Medicine PCotASfR. Role of metformin for ovulation induction in infertile patients with polycystic ovary syndrome (PCOS): a guideline. *Fertility and Sterility.* 2017;108(3):426-41.

[248] Kalem M, Kalem Z, Gurgan T. Effect of metformin and oral contraceptives on polycystic ovary syndrome and IVF cycles. *Journal of Endocrinological Investigation.* 2017;40(7):745-52.

[249] Wu Y, Tu M, Huang Y, Liu Y, Zhang D. Association of metformin with pregnancy outcomes in women with polycystic ovarian

syndrome undergoing in vitro fertilization: A systematic review and meta-analysis. *JAMA network open.* 2020;3(8):e2011995-e.

[250] Hashim HA. Twenty years of ovulation induction with metformin for PCOS; what is the best available evidence? *Reproductive biomedicine online.* 2016;32(1):44-53.

[251] Magee P, Pearson S, Whittingham-Dowd J, Allen J. PPARγ as a molecular target of EPA anti-inflammatory activity during TNF-α-impaired skeletal muscle cell differentiation. *The Journal of nutritional biochemistry.* 2012;23(11):1440-8.

[252] Mohammadi E, Rafraf M, Farzadi L, Asghari-Jafarabadi M, Sabour S. Effects of omega-3 fatty acids supplementation on serum adiponectin levels and some metabolic risk factors in women with polycystic ovary syndrome. *Asia Pacific journal of clinical nutrition.* 2012;21(4):511.

[253] Yang K, Zeng L, Bao T, Ge J. Effectiveness of omega-3 fatty acid for polycystic ovary syndrome: a systematic review and meta-analysis. *Reproductive Biology and Endocrinology.* 2018;16(1):27.

[254] Oner G, Muderris I. Efficacy of omega-3 in the treatment of polycystic ovary syndrome. *Journal of Obstetrics and Gynaecology.* 2013;33(3):289-91.

[255] Tosatti JA, Alves MT, Cândido AL, Reis FM, Araújo VE, Gomes KB. Influence of n-3 fatty acid supplementation on inflammatory and oxidative stress markers in patients with polycystic ovary syndrome: a systematic review and meta-analysis. *British Journal of Nutrition.* 2020:1-12.

[256] Mirmasoumi G, Fazilati M, Foroozanfard F, Vahedpoor Z, Mahmoodi S, Taghizadeh M, et al. The effects of flaxseed oil omega-3 fatty acids supplementation on metabolic status of patients with polycystic ovary syndrome: a randomized, double-blind, placebo-controlled trial. *Experimental and clinical endocrinology & diabetes.* 2018;126(04):222-8.

[257] Haidari F, Banaei-Jahromi N, Zakerkish M, Ahmadi K. The effects of flaxseed supplementation on metabolic status in women with

polycystic ovary syndrome: a randomized open-labeled controlled clinical trial. *Nutrition Journal.* 2020;19(1):8.

[258] Bareksei A, Hafner G, Pfeiffer S, Schlatterer K. Effects of Periconceptual Omega-3-Fatty Acid Supplementation on in Vitro Fertilization Success and Miscarriage Rates in Patients of a German Fertility Centre. *International Journal of Clinical and Experimental Medical Sciences.* 2019;5(5):62.

[259] Vahed MG, Khanbabaee R, Shariati M, Edalatmanesh MA. Improving the Effects of Omega-3 Fatty Acid on the In Vitro Maturation of Oocytes. *Jurnal Ilmu Ternak dan Veteriner.* 2020;25(4):153-61.

[260] Rashidi B, Abediasl J, Tehraninejad E, Rahmanpour H, Sills ES. Simvastatin effects on androgens, inflammatory mediators, and endogenous pituitary gonadotropins among patients with PCOS undergoing IVF: results from a prospective, randomized, placebo-controlled clinical trial. *Journal of Investigative Medicine.* 2011;59(6):912-6.

[261] Banaszewska B, Pawelczyk L, Spaczynski RZ, Duleba AJ. Effects of simvastatin and metformin on polycystic ovary syndrome after six months of treatment. *The Journal of Clinical Endocrinology & Metabolism.* 2011;96(11):3493-501.

[262] Duleba AJ, Banaszewska B, Spaczynski RZ, Pawelczyk L. Simvastatin improves biochemical parameters in women with polycystic ovary syndrome: results of a prospective, randomized trial. *Fertility and Sterility.* 2006;85(4):996-1001.

[263] Celik O, Acbay O. Effects of metformin plus rosuvastatin on hyperandrogenism in polycystic ovary syndrome patients with hyperlipidemia and impaired glucose tolerance. *Journal of Endocrinological Investigation.* 2012;35(10):905-10.

[264] Gao L, Zhao FL, Li SC. Statin is a reasonable treatment option for patients with polycystic ovary syndrome: a meta-analysis of randomized controlled trials. *Experimental and clinical endocrinology & diabetes.* 2012;120(06):367-75.

[265] Kazerooni T, Shojaei-Baghini A, Dehbashi S, Asadi N, Ghaffarpasand F, Kazerooni Y. Effects of metformin plus simvastatin on polycystic ovary syndrome: a prospective, randomized, double-blind, placebo-controlled study. *Fertility and Sterility*. 2010;94 (6):2208-13.

[266] Raja-Khan N, Kunselman AR, Hogeman CS, Stetter CM, Demers LM, Legro RS. Effects of atorvastatin on vascular function, inflammation, and androgens in women with polycystic ovary syndrome: a double-blind, randomized, placebo-controlled trial. *Fertility and Sterility*. 2011;95(5):1849-52.

[267] Puurunen J, Piltonen T, Puukka K, Ruokonen A, Savolainen MJ, Bloigu R, et al. Statin therapy worsens insulin sensitivity in women with polycystic ovary syndrome (PCOS): a prospective, randomized, double-blind, placebo-controlled study. *The Journal of Clinical Endocrinology & Metabolism*. 2013;98(12):4798-807.

[268] Sun J, Yuan Y, Cai R, Sun H, Zhou Y, Wang P, et al. An investigation into the therapeutic effects of statins with metformin on polycystic ovary syndrome: a meta-analysis of randomised controlled trials. *BMJ open*. 2015;5(3).

[269] Seyam E, Al Gelany S, Abd Al Ghaney A, Mohamed MAA, Youseff AM, Ibrahim EM, et al. Evaluation of prolonged use of statins on the clinical and biochemical abnormalities and ovulation dysfunction in single young women with polycystic ovary syndrome. *Gynecological Endocrinology*. 2018;34(7):589-96.

[270] Seyam E, Hefzy E. Long-term effects of combined simvastatin and metformin treatment on the clinical abnormalities and ovulation dysfunction in single young women with polycystic ovary syndrome. *Gynecological Endocrinology*. 2018;34(12):1073-80.

[271] Meng J, Zhu Y. Efficacy of simvastatin plus metformin for polycystic ovary syndrome: a meta-analysis of randomized controlled trials. *European Journal of Obstetrics & Gynecology and Reproductive Biology*. 2020.

[272] Ramírez-Garza SL, Laveriano-Santos EP, Marhuenda-Muñoz M, Storniolo CE, Tresserra-Rimbau A, Vallverdú-Queralt A, et al. Health

effects of resveratrol: Results from human intervention trials. *Nutrients.* 2018;10(12):1892.

[273] Wong DH, Villanueva JA, Cress AB, Sokalska A, Ortega I, Duleba AJ. Resveratrol inhibits the mevalonate pathway and potentiates the antiproliferative effects of simvastatin in rat theca-interstitial cells. *Fertility and Sterility.* 2011;96(5):1252-8.

[274] Zhu X, Wu C, Qiu S, Yuan X, Li L. Effects of resveratrol on glucose control and insulin sensitivity in subjects with type 2 diabetes: Systematic review and meta-analysis. *Nutrition & metabolism.* 2017;14(1):60.

[275] Banaszewska B Ws-BsJ, Spaczynski RZ, Pawelczyk L, Duleba AJ. Effects of resveratrol on polycystic ovary syndrome: a double-blind, randomized, placebo-controlled trial. *J Clin Endocrinol Metab.* 2016;101(11):4322-8.

[276] Ortega I, de la Fuente AA, Matey S, Henzenn E, Cruz M, Pacheco A, et al. Resveratrol for Preventing Ovarian Hyperstimulation Syndrome in Women at Risk Undergoing Egg Donation: A Randomized Controlled Study. *Fertility and Sterility.* 2020;114(3):e454.

[277] Brenjian S, Moini A, Yamini N, Kashani L, Faridmojtahedi M, Bahramrezaie M, et al. Resveratrol treatment in patients with polycystic ovary syndrome decreased pro-inflammatory and endoplasmic reticulum stress markers. *American Journal of Reproductive Immunology.* 2020;83(1):e13186.

[278] Kim CH, Chon SJ, Lee SH. Effects of lifestyle modification in polycystic ovary syndrome compared to metformin only or metformin addition: A systematic review and meta-analysis. *Scientific reports.* 2020;10(1):1-13.

[279] Moran L, Hutchison S, Norman R, Teede H. *Lifestyle Changes in Women With Polycystic Ovary Syndrome: Cochrane Database of Systematic Reviews.* Hoboken, NJ: Wiley-Blackwell; 2011.

[280] Pasquali R. Lifestyle Interventions and Natural and Assisted Reproduction in Patients with PCOS. *Infertility in Women with Polycystic Ovary Syndrome*: Springer; 2018. p. 169-80.

[281] Li Y-m, Hu S, He F, Liu D. *Effect of different levels of weight loss on clinical outcomes in obese women with polycystic ovary syndrome underwent assisted reproduction.* 2020.

[282] Moran L, Tsagareli V, Norman R, Noakes M. Diet and IVF pilot study: short-term weight loss improves pregnancy rates in overweight/obese women undertaking IVF. *Australian and New Zealand Journal of Obstetrics and Gynaecology.* 2011;51(5):455-9.

[283] Becker GF, Passos EP, Moulin CC. Short-term effects of a hypocaloric diet with low glycemic index and low glycemic load on body adiposity, metabolic variables, ghrelin, leptin, and pregnancy rate in overweight and obese infertile women: a randomized controlled trial. *The American journal of clinical nutrition.* 2015;102(6):1365-72.

[284] Alibeigi Z, Jafari-Dehkordi E, Kheiri S, Nemati M, Mohammadi-Farsani G, Tansaz M. The Impact of Traditional Medicine-Based Lifestyle and Diet on Infertility Treatment in Women Undergoing Assisted Reproduction: A Randomized Controlled Trial. *Complementary Medicine Research.* 2020:1-12.

[285] Van Oers AM, Mutsaerts MA, Burggraaff JM, Kuchenbecker WK, Perquin DA, Koks CA, et al. Cost-effectiveness analysis of lifestyle intervention in obese infertile women. *Human reproduction.* 2017;32(7):1418-26.

[286] Moran LJ, Noakes M, Clifton PM, Tomlinson L, Norman RJ. Dietary composition in restoring reproductive and metabolic physiology in overweight women with polycystic ovary syndrome. *The Journal of Clinical Endocrinology & Metabolism.* 2003;88(2):812-9.

[287] Moini A, Arabipoor A, Hemat M, Ahmadi J, Salman-Yazdi R, Zolfaghari Z. The effect of weight loss program on serum anti-Müllerian hormone level in obese and overweight infertile women with polycystic ovary syndrome. *Gynecological Endocrinology.* 2019;35(2):119-23.

[288] Salama AA, Amine EK, Salem HAE, Abd El Fattah NK. Anti-inflammatory dietary combo in overweight and obese women with

polycystic ovary syndrome. *North American journal of medical sciences.* 2015;7(7):310.

[289] Sears B, Ricordi C. Anti-inflammatory nutrition as a pharmacological approach to treat obesity. *Journal of Obesity.* 2011;2011.

[290] Salama AA, Amine E, Hesham A, Abd El-Fatteh N. Effects of anti-inflammatory diet in the context of lifestyle modification (with or without metformin use) on metabolic, endocrine, inflammatory and reproductive profiles in overweight and obese women with polycystic ovary syndrome: Controlled clinical trial. *Canadian Journal of Clinical Nutrition.* 2018;6:81-106.

In: Polycystic Ovary Syndrome
Editor: Katherine Webb
ISBN: 978-1-53619-527-9
© 2021 Nova Science Publishers, Inc.

Chapter 2

AN OVERVIEW OF POSSIBLE HEALTH RISK AND COMPLICATIONS OF POLYCYSTIC OVARY SYNDROME

Iram Ashaq Kawa[1], Akbar Masood[1], Shahnaz Ahmad Mir[2], Saika Manzoor[1] and Fouzia Rashid[1]

[1]Department of Biochemistry/Clinical Biochemistry, University of Kashmir, Srinagar, Jammu and Kashmir, India
[2]Department of Endocrinology, Government Medical College, Shireen Bagh, Srinagar, Jammu and Kashmir, India

ABSTRACT

Polycystic Ovary Syndrome (PCOS) is the most common disorder associated with a spectrum of endocrine, reproductive, metabolic and psychological features. It affects millions of women worldwide and represents a major burden on health and economy. PCOS women are usually diagnosed in adolescence or in early adulthood with signs of hirsutism, acne or oligomenorrhea or when presenting for treatment of infertility. However, the health issues associated with PCOS go well beyond the management of these typical symptoms and likely persist throughout the reproductive years and beyond menopause which significantly affects the quality of life of these women. Amidst its prevalence and repercussions for metabolic, reproductive and psychological wellbeing PCOS remains under-diagnosed; partly because of the heterogeneity of the phenotypes presented by the syndrome. The phenotypes vary significantly depending on the stage of life, ethnicity, genotype and environmental factors like Body Mass Index and lifestyle. Although the pathogenesis of this syndrome remains elusive, abnormalities in action or secretion of gonadotropin, steroidogenesis, folliculogenesis, insulin action or secretion among others contribute to its development. The dysregulation of these diverse systems is thought to result from genetic, epigenetic and environmental factors. A better understanding of these factors is important for the determination of preventive risk factors and effective treatment of this syndrome. The primary concern of this complex disorder is timely diagnosis; education of patients and healthcare professionals; screening and treatment for complications that would reduce the health and economic burden associated with PCOS and its related co-morbid conditions. Keeping in view the complexity of this syndrome and the impact on the quality of life of these women, this chapter will try to shed some light on the clinical presentation, diagnosis and pathogenesis of PCOS. This chapter will also present a general overview on complications and associated health risks of this syndrome.

INTRODUCTION

Polycystic Ovary Syndrome

Polycystic Ovary Syndrome (PCOS) is the most common endocrine disorder of reproductive age women with a global prevalence of 6 to 20% depending on the diagnostic criteria used to define the syndrome [1]. The term "polycystic ovarian syndrome" does not entirely or accurately reflect the disorder's nature owing to its very wide range of clinical manifestations and related morbidities. Stein and Leventhal are regarded to have been the first to describe PCOS in 1935 as gynecological disorder, when seven women presented with menstrual disturbances, hirsutism (a condition of male pattern terminal hair growth in women) and bilateral polycystic ovaries [2]. However, it was in 1721 when Italian scientist Vallisneri described for the first time a young married, infertile and moderately obese woman with shiny white ovaries, and the size of pigeon eggs [3]. Then it was not until the early 1990s that a formal diagnostic criterion for PCOS was introduced at a conference held by National Institute of Health (NIH) [4]. It is now recognized as a complex disorder with a broad spectrum of manifestations affecting the endocrine, metabolic and reproductive functions of such women thus leading to decreased quality of life.

Definition and Prevalence

Over the past three decades three diagnostic criteria have been proposed for PCOS as shown in Table 1. The National Institute of Child Health and Human Development of the US National Institutes of Health (NIH) conference first attempted to classify PCOS in April 1990. The NIH criteria, requires both clinical hyperandrogenism and/or biochemical hyperandrogenemia, together with chronic oligo-/anovulation to be present [4]. In 2003, the European Society of Human Reproduction and Embryology/American Society for Reproductive Medicine Rotterdam consensus (ESHRE/ASRM) meeting was held by 27 PCOS experts in Rotterdam, the Netherlands. The Rotterdam criteria introduced the third criterion, the appearance of polycystic ovaries by ultrasound and requires the presence of two of the three features: oligo-/anovulation (defined as >35-day cycle or mid luteal progesterone <2.5 ng/mL), clinical and/or biochemical hyperandrogenism (defined as acne, hirsutism or elevated free or total testosterone levels and ultrasonographic ovarian morphology (defined as >10 mL ovarian volume, or >12 follicles measuring 2–9 mm in at least one ovary) [5]. The change brought by Rotterdam criteria by inclusion of polycystic ovaries has led to the identification of PCOS as a disorder with varied number of complex clinical phenotypes and varying outcomes. In 2006, the Androgen Excess and PCOS Society (AE-PCOS) criteria was introduced and according to AE-PCOS criteria, PCOS is a condition primarily of androgen excess and therefore diagnosis should be based on the presence of hyperandrogenism plus ovarian dysfunction and/or polycystic ovaries, reducing the number of phenotypic possibilities [6]. Each of these criteria considers PCOS a diagnosis of exclusion, and excluding other diagnoses such as non-classic adrenal hyperplasia, congenital adrenal hyperplasia, Cushing syndrome, androgen-secreting tumor, hyperprolactinemia, idiopathic hirsutism, idiopathic hyperandrogenism, drug-induced androgen excess and thyroid disorders. Twelve years later, due to controversies between diagnostic criteria, NIH sponsored Evidence-based Methodology Workshop (NIH and ESHRE/ASRM) on PCOS in 2012 recommended the wider Rotterdam/ESHRE/ASRM 2003 criteria together with the phenotyping specifications as 1) hyperandrogenism (Clinical and/or biochemical) plus ovulatory dysfunction (oligo- or anovulation); 2) hyperandrogenism plus Polycystic Ovary Morphology (PCOM); 3) hyperandrogenism plus ovulatory dysfunction plus PCOM; 4) ovulatory dysfunction plus PCOM [7]. Presently out of various diagnostic criteria of PCOS, the Rotterdam criterion is found to be more inclusive and most commonly used.

Different prevalence estimates of PCOS were identified by various studies when three sets of diagnostic criteria known as NIH, Rotterdam and AE-PCOS criteria are applied. The highest prevalence is seen when the feature of polycystic ovaries is included in the diagnosis. The worldwide prevalence of PCOS across most of these studies has been relatively uniform between 5 and 10% defined by NIH criteria, 5 to 20% by Rotterdam criteria and prevalence ranges from 10-15% by AE-PCOS criteria [8]. There are only few studies available regarding the prevalence of PCOS among Indian women. A study conducted among young Indian women aged between 18-24 years by Nidhi et al., reported a prevalence of 9.1% by NIH criteria [9]. A study conducted by Nair et al., among adolescents showed a prevalence of 36% by Rotterdam criteria [10]. An urban community-based study conducted by Joshi et al., reported a prevalence of 22.5% by the Rotterdam criteria and 10.7% by the AE-PCOS criteria [11]. In Kashmir valley also a cross-sectional pilot study was conducted among women of reproductive age across educational institutions to estimate the prevalence of PCOS. The Prevalence was reported to be higher than other Asian communities as 28.9% by the NIH criteria, 35.3% by the Rotterdam criteria and 34.3% by the AE-PCOS criteria [12]. These variations among the studies using the same diagnostic criteria across countries might be due to population of different ethnicity/race, geographical factors, and differences in the characteristics of the study population, difficulties in phenotypic interpretation and design limitations.

Table 1: Diagnostic criteria for polycystic ovary syndrome (PCOS)

	Diagnostic criteria for PCOS	
NIH (1990)	**Rotterdam (2003)**	**Androgen Excess Society (2006)**
Requires both	Requires 2 out of 3	Requires both
Clinical and/or Biochemical signs of Hyperandrogenism	Clinical and/or Biochemical signs of Hyperandrogenism	Clinical and/or Biochemical signs of Hyperandrogenism
Oligo-anovulation	Oligo-anovulation	Oligo-anovulation and/or Polycystic Ovaries on USG
	Polycystic Ovaries on USG	
All criteria require exclusion of other related disorders such as congenital adrenal hyperplasia, non-classic adrenal hyperplasia, Cushing syndrome, androgen-secreting tumor, idiopathic hyperandrogenism, idiopathic hirsutism, hyperprolactinemia, and thyroid disorders.		
Abbreviations: PCOS, Polycystic Ovary Syndrome; NIH, National Institute of Health; USG, Ultrasonography.		

Clinical Manifestations of PCOS

PCOS is a heterogeneous disorder which affects not only the reproductive age women but also adolescents and postmenopausal women. It is mostly characterized by clinical or biochemical hyperandrogenism, oligo anovulation and polycystic ovarian morphology which we define as follows and is depicted in Figure 1:

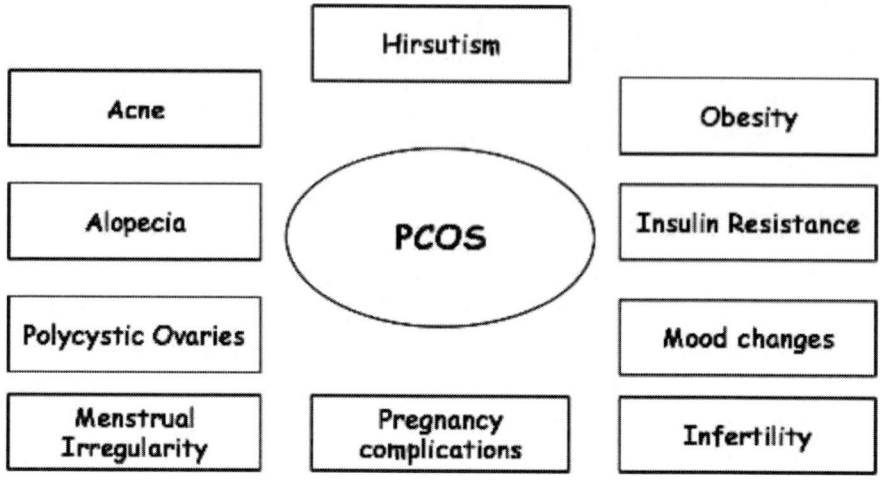

Figure 1. Clinical Presentation of Polycystic Ovary Syndrome (PCOS).

Hyperandrogenism

Hyperandrogenism or androgen excess is a common endocrine disorder affecting about 7% of reproductive age women and approximately 80 to 85% women with androgen excess have PCOS [13, 14]. It is one of the hallmark features of PCOS pathophysiology. Androgens are primarily produced by ovaries and adrenal glands; peripheral tissues including fat and skin also play a role in transforming androgens into more potent forms. Hyperandrogen diagnosis can be based on clinical symptoms or excess serum androgen measurements. The clinical manifestations can be observed even when the biochemical hyperandrogenism is not present. It is observed that about 70% of PCOS women have moderately elevated free testosterone and 20-30% have mildly elevated dehydroepiandrosterone sulphate (DHEAS). Clinically it manifests as hirsutism, seborrhea (oily skin), acne, androgenic alopecia, menstrual irregularity, infertility, weight gain, subcutaneous and abdominal fat among others [15]. The extent of clinical hyperandrogenic presentation varies between individuals and is influenced by many factors, including genetic polymorphism, inadequate epigenetic reprogramming, metabolism and other environmental factors.

Hirsutism

Hirsutism is the primary clinical marker of androgen excess and is defined as the male pattern excessive terminal hair growth (body and facial) at androgen dependent areas in women. Approximately 70-80% of hirsute women have hyperandrogenism and about 70% of PCOS women have hirsutism which varies with race and obesity [7, 16]. The severity and extent of hirsutism is assessed by using a standard scoring system known as modified Ferriman-Gallwey hirsutism score in which nine body parts (upper lip, chin, chest, upper back, lower back, upper abdomen, lower abdomen, arm, and thigh) are evaluated for the presence of hair growth between 0 (no visible terminal hairs) and 4 (extensive growth of terminal hairs) and a score of > 8 out of a total of 36 is taken as significant [17, 18]. The presence of excessive hair growth results in psychological morbidity and adversely affects the quality of life of such women.

Seborrhea

Seborrhea or oily skin is another cutaneous manifestation of PCOS and its prevalence in PCOS is not exactly known. It is characterized by the presence of greasy or shiny skin on the forehead, the nasolabial folds, or behind the ear and scalp which occurs due to the increased production of sebum by oversized sebaceous glands. It is often followed by large pores and results in the formation of acne [19]. The sebaceous gland is a target organ of androgen and enhanced activity of sebaceous gland is due to the potent androgen 5α-dihydrotestosterone. Sebaceous gland cells have all the required enzymes to transform testosterone to 5α-dihydrotestosterone (5α-DHT). The type 1 isoenzyme 5α-reductase catalyzes the conversion of testosterone to 5α-dihydrotestosterone in peripheral tissues and is predominantly expressed in skin.

Both testosterone and 5α-dihydrotestosterone mediate their function by binding to nuclear androgen receptors (AR) which is also expressed in sebaceous gland cells. However, the affinity for AR is more for 5α-dihydrotestosterone and 5α-DHT/AR complex tends to be more stable and thus, more efficient [20]. Apart from androgens, seborrhea is also influenced by age, gender, genetic predisposition, ethnicity and climate. For this reason, clinical, biochemical and radiological examinations for the diagnosis of PCOS-related seborrhea are significant.

Acne

Acne is a common and most frequently encountered dermatological condition known to affect more than 80% of adolescents and it continues throughout adulthood [21]. Females are more affected than males with a prevalence of 15% in all age group [22, 23]. It is of multifactorial etiology and results from the combination of increased activity of sebaceous gland, abnormal follicular epithelial differentiation, hypercolonization of microbes in follicle canal, increased inflammation and genetic elements among others [24]. Androgens are also known to play a significant role in its pathogenesis [25]. However, the association of acne with androgen excess is not completely understood and is debatable. Nevertheless, androgens stimulate the proliferation of sebocyte increasing the sebum production and also results in the formation of comedones (black heads and white heads) by abnormal desquamation of follicular epithelial cells. It is characterized by inflammatory lesions like pustules, papules, nobless, nodules, cysts and non-inflammatory lesions- white heads and black heads [26]. A number of systems are employed to assess the grading severity of acne. In general acne severity is evaluated by the number, form and distribution of the lesions [27]. Acne is one of the cutaneous manifestations of PCOS and is reported to be present in 15 to 30% of PCOS women [28].

The prevalence of acne alone i.e., without hirsutism is very less in these women and is mostly present on facial area with 50% women involving other body parts as well like neck, chest and upper back. While the exclusive presence of acne is a potential marker of hyperandrogenism, it is clear that patients with acne do not have excess androgen and data on prevalence of hyperandrogenism in these patients are scarce [29, 30]. Therefore, the sole presence of acne might not be considered as hyperandrogenic sign. However in women with severe acne or associated with hirsutism or menstrual irregularity, hyperandrogenism should be considered.

Alopecia

Alopecia in women refers to the male pattern hair loss and is an extremely stressful condition with substantially deleterious impact on self-esteem, mood, body image and overall quality of life. While women have multiple causes of alopecia which include autoimmune disorders, infections, neoplasm and trauma, androgenic alopecia is the most common form. Androgenic alopecia or more recently known as female pattern hair loss is the most common cause of alopecia in women. It is seen in 10% of PCOS patients and is characterized by the loss of hair density primarily on vertex (top) and frontal regions of scalp or in a diffused pattern. There is no complete baldness in women with androgenic alopecia as seen in men however, in these areas the hair becomes thinner and shorter and the hair follicle remains alive. The biological hair follicle cycle is divided into three phases: anagen (growth phase), catagen (regression) and telogen (resting phase). The original hair falls out at the end of resting phase i.e., telogen phase and is replaced by a new hair at the early stage of growth. The underlying mechanism for scalp hair thinning in androgenic alopecia are miniaturization of hair follicles and decreased length of hair cycle growth phase i.e., anagen phase leading to an increased proportion of telogen hair.

There is also a delay between the end of the telogen phase and the start of new anagen phase leading to an overall decrease in scalp hair shafts [31]. Moreover, there may be some role of ethnicity and familial inheritance pattern of androgenic alopecia. Alopecia is commonly graded using the classification system of Ludwig, which classifies the pattern into three degrees from first degree with mild light thinning to the third degree with total absence of hair in the affected area [32].

Ovarian Dysfunction

Ovarian dysfunction is the most common feature of PCOS and usually presents as oligomenorrhea or amenorrhea, resulting from chronic oligo-ovulation/anovulation. It is generally not accompanied by premenstrual symptoms like bloating, mood changes and tenderness of the breasts indicating anovulation. Oligomenorrhea is defined as the infrequent cycles with the occurrence of menstrual cycles greater than 35 days apart and amenorrhea is the absence of menstrual cycles for three or more months. Ovarian dysfunction is observed in approximately 70 to 80% of PCOS women. It is also reported that about 85 to 90% of women with oligomenorrhea will have PCOS and 30 to 40% of amenorrheic women will have PCOS [28]. Some women may present ovarian dysfunction as polymenorrhoea in which the menstrual cycle length is less than 21 days. It is, however, possible to have ovulatory dysfunction even with normal cycle especially in women with clinical signs of androgen excess and can be demonstrated by measuring the serum progesterone levels during luteal phase of menstrual cycle. The main clinical manifestation of ovulatory dysfunction in PCOS is infertility. About 75% of PCOS patients present with anovulatory infertility making PCOS the most common cause of anovulatory infertility [33]. Obesity further accelerates the infertility and studies have shown that obese PCOS patients have more ovulation impairments and lower rates of pregnancy than the normal weight PCOS women.

Polycystic Ovarian Morphology

While Polycystic Ovarian Morphology (PCOM) can be confirmed histopathologically, clinically transvaginal ultrasonography detects most of the polycystic ovarian morphology. The most commonly used Rotterdam criteria defines PCOM as the presence of 12 or more follicles measuring 2 to 9 millimeters in size per ovary or ovary volume greater than 10mL or both [5]. However, with the advancement in ultrasonography machinery the diagnosis of PCOM was updated and defined as the presence of 25 follicles or more rather than 12 per ovary (only when ≥8 MHz transducer frequency used) or ovary volume 10mL or more (when <8 MHz transducer frequency used), or both [34].

PCOS and its Associated Morbidities

There is a plethora of health problems associated with PCOS diagnosis, many of which represent complications for a lifetime. PCOS is associated with metabolic aberrations such as insulin resistance, obesity and dyslipidemia contributing to increased lifetime risk of developing cardiovascular diseases, type 2 diabetes mellitus, hypertension and psychological features like anxiety, depression, poor self-esteem, eating disorders and psychosexual dysfunction. PCOS is also associated with pregnancy complications like gestational diabetes, pre-eclampsia, fetal macrosomia, small-for-gestational age infants and perinatal mortality. Therefore, the impact of this disorder is not limited to the reproductive age, but continues throughout life.

Metabolic Aberrations

One of the most prevalent risks involves metabolic abnormalities and their associated manifestations which are discussed below and shown in Figure 2.

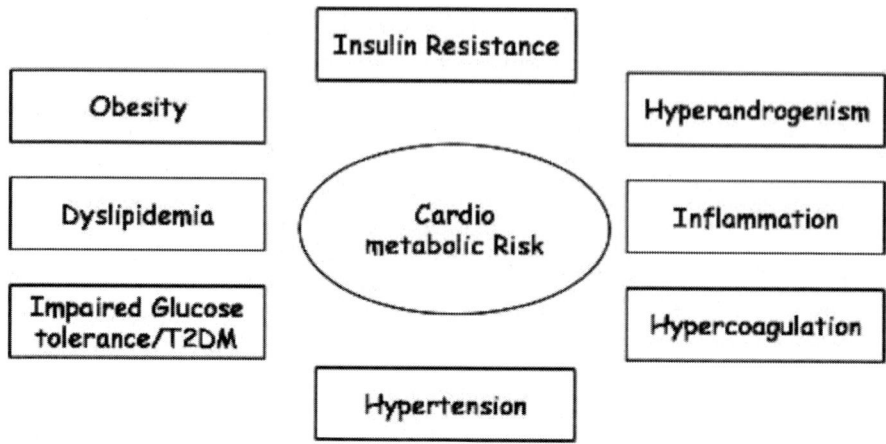

Figure 2. Cardiometabolic risk factors in Polycystic Ovary Syndrome (PCOS).

Obesity

The prevalence of obesity has increased globally in recent decades and reached a pandemic proportion [35]. In developing countries approximately one-third of adults are obese and one-third are overweight. This increase in the obesity prevalence has significant health care consequences, as obesity is a significant risk factor for cardiovascular diseases and all-cause mortality, not limited to adult population. In addition to its cardiometabolic complications obesity is strongly associated with PCOS. It is the common characteristic feature among PCOS women. About 50% of women with PCOS are overweight or obese and often have abdominal phenotype. The history of weight gain often comes prior to the onset of hyperandrogenism and oligomenorrhea, signifying the etiologic role of obesity in the subsequent development of the syndrome. There are also mechanisms, however, wherein PCOS development may lead to further weight gain and can impede efforts to achieve successful weight loss, thereby creating a vicious cycle that can be hard to overcome [36]. Obesity, especially visceral adiposity that is common in obese and non-obese women with PCOS, amplifies and exacerbates all PCOS metabolic and reproductive outcomes. It may in part be responsible for insulin resistance and subsequent hyperinsulinemia in PCOS women. PCOS women are at higher risk for metabolic syndrome and cardiovascular risk that are linked to insulin resistance including dyslipidemia and type 2 diabetes. Obese PCOS patients appear to have higher risks of metabolic disorders, characterized by elevated levels of lipid profile, fasting glucose and insulin resistance [37]. Obesity also has an impact on hyperandrogenism in PCOS women and there are consistent evidences that demonstrate the increased body weight in PCOS women favor a deteriorated hyperandrogenic condition. Obesity also has greater impact on female fertility which includes irregular menstrual cycles, impaired ovulation, increased rate of miscarriage and poor pregnancy outcomes among others. Hence, obesity appears to worsen the PCOS reproductive and metabolic phenotype. Further, it is shown that the prevalence of PCOS in overweight/obese women is substantially increased regardless of the existence of the metabolic syndrome, indicating that all premenopausal overweight/obese patients seeking weight loss should be screened for PCOS regardless of their metabolic profile, in order to treat or alleviate the health burden associated with this prevalent syndrome [38]. Waist circumference, body mass index and waist hip ratio are the surrogate indicators of obesity, in particular waist circumference for visceral adiposity.

Insulin Resistance

Insulin resistance is defined as a condition of a cell, tissue or organism that requires increased amount of insulin to obtain the appropriate response. The increased secretion of insulin by pancreatic β-cells leads to compensatory hyperinsulinemia. As long as insulin resistance is overcome by hyperinsulinemia, levels of glucose remain normal. As β-cells decline in compensatory response, it results in relative or absolute insulin insufficiency with metabolic consequences. In addition to metabolic effects insulin performs both mitogenic and reproductive actions. Insulin resistance is a distinctive feature of PCOS that occurs in 50-70% of PCOS women independent of obesity, though it's not universal and varies between PCOS clinical phenotypes [39, 40]. About 90% of obese PCOS women have insulin resistance and its effect is additive to that of PCOS [41]. Long-term worsening of insulin resistance may be a significant factor in the development of glucose intolerance states (including impaired glucose tolerance, type 2 diabetes, gestational diabetes) in women with PCOS, especially in the presence of obesity [42]. This rarely happens in those with average weight, indicating obesity may reflect a critical prerequisite. Insulin resistance in PCOS also leads to hyperandrogenism and anovulation [43]. Interestingly in PCOS the "key anomaly" is that ovaries remain susceptible to the action of insulin to produce androgens despite the systemic state of insulin resistance. The molecular mechanism resulting in insulin resistance in PCOS remains unclear. Genetic factors, epigenetic changes, extra-uterine environmental effects, prenatal exposures, and inconsistent nutrient excess adaptations likely lead to insulin resistance development and hyperinsulinemia. Homeostatic model assessment, fasting glucose-to-insulin ratio, and quantitative insulin sensitivity check index are currently used as surrogate markers of insulin resistance in clinical research and practice because of the complexity and cost of gold standard hyperinsulinemia euglycemic clamp technique for insulin resistance diagnosis [44]. Clinically insulin resistance may present as Acanthosis nigricans which is a skin lesion characterized by the thickened, dark, velvety, hyperkeratotic, hyperpigmented, papillomatous skin patches around neck, groin, antecubital fossae, in the axillae or in areas under the breast and in other skin folds [45]. It occurs in extreme hyperinsulinemia and hyperandrogenism. Hyperandrogenism, insulin resistance and acanthosis nigricans together constitute an unusual condition that affects females known as hyperandrogenic insulin-resistant acanthosis nigricans (HAIR-AN) syndrome and should be excluded when considering a diagnosis of PCOS [46].

Dyslipidemia

Dyslipidemia is one of the most frequently seen metabolic aberrations among PCOS women. About 70% of PCOS women have dyslipidemia [47]. Even though there are discrepancies in the form and degree of lipid abnormalities, hypertriglyceridemia, low HDL (high density lipoprotein) cholesterol concentration, high LDL (low density lipoprotein) cholesterol levels are typical features among the definitions of dyslipidemia and emerges as a significant risk factor for cardiovascular diseases [48]. In PCOS the cause of dyslipidemia is multifactorial; insulin resistance seems to have a significant role partly mediated by stimulation of lipolysis and altered lipoprotein lipase and hepatic lipase expression [48]. Dyslipidemia occurs independently of BMI; however, obesity and insulin resistance have synergistic deleterious effect on PCOS similar to that of type 2 diabetes [49]. The waist to hip ratio, higher among women with PCOS is susceptible to dyslipidemia as central adipocytes appear to have an adverse effect on blood lipids. It is because central fat is more insulin resistant and generates fatty acids faster by lipolysis as compared to the peripheral fat [50]. Recent guidelines recommend a complete lipid profile (triglycerides, total cholesterol, HDL cholesterol and LDL cholesterol) for all PCOS women, regardless of age as part of assessment of their cardiovascular risk.

Impaired Glucose Tolerance and Type 2 Diabetes

Women with PCOS present with substantially increased prevalence of Impaired Glucose Tolerance (IGT) and Type 2 Diabetes Mellitus (T2DM) independent of BMI as compared to weight matched healthy women. Recent meta-analysis studies have shown a 2.5-fold increased prevalence of IGT and 4-fold increased prevalence of T2DM in PCOS women compared to women without PCOS, independent of obesity and appears higher with obesity [42, 51]. A follow up study of 10 years showed the age-standardized prevalence of T2DM in the age of 40s and 50s in PCOS women is 40%, which is 6.8 times more than that of similar age general female population [52]. Insulin resistance, a significant metabolic burden present in both obese and lean PCOS women has been recognized as the main risk factor of T2DM development and is likely to contribute to high prevalence of IGT in PCOS women [53]. PCOS women often experience impaired glucose metabolism at an early age and can exhibit a faster transition from IGT to T2DM [54]. Obesity and family history of diabetes among young and middle aged PCOS women further increases their risk of developing diabetes. In addition to converting to IGT/T2DM, PCOS women also present a high risk of developing gestational diabetes mellitus, independent of obesity and are exacerbated by it [55]. Because diabetes is one of the leading cause of mortality and morbidity, screening of high risk women with T2DM such as women with pre-diabetes, obesity, insulin resistance and PCOS is important.

Oral glucose tolerance test is suggested to be the best screening tool for measuring glucose intolerance and diabetes in PCOS women as most women with PCOS and glucose intolerance were previously reported to have normal fasting glucose levels [53]. Early detection, lifestyle modification and pharmacological treatment may help to delay the progression of IGT to T2DM.

Cardiovascular Disease

Women with PCOS clearly show a higher risk of developing cardiovascular diseases in adult life due to their unusual hormonal pattern and associated metabolic aberrations described by hyperandrogenism, insulin resistance, obesity, dyslipidemia, diabetes, hypertension and inflammatory condition. In addition to these very well-known risk factors for cardiovascular disease, other markers of cardiovascular disease are also found to be increased in PCOS women like homocysteine and C reactive protein [56]. Also, early subclinical and clinical atherosclerosis markers are observed in PCOS women which are further worsened by obesity such as increased carotid intima media wall thickness, endothelial dysfunction, elevated artery calcification and presence of carotid plaque compared to controls [55]. Many studies and meta-analysis have shown higher risk of coronary heart disease and stroke in PCOS women compared to women without PCOS. Further, studies have shown that an increased risk of cardiovascular disease in both obese and non-obese PCOS women is related to higher severity of PCOS phenotypes [57, 58]. Many studies have demonstrated an increased cardiovascular disease risk in PCOS women, but these results are not universal. Few other studies on the other hand, reported no statistically significant relation between PCOS and related cardiovascular consequences. In view of this disparity and limited long-term studies to appropriately address the risk of cardiovascular disease in PCOS, more population based long term studies assessing the impact of cardiovascular disease risk factors and associated cardiovascular consequences are needed to enhance our knowledge of the implications of risk factors on PCOS women. This will effectively guide strategies and interventions to reduce the risk of cardiovascular disease for these women.

Psychological Implications

Apart from the evident reproductive endocrinologic and metabolic aberrations, there are also serious psychological repercussions. This might be due to the symptoms like acne, hirsutism, alopecia and others which would make PCOS women feel the loss of feminine traits and attractiveness thus decreases their self-esteem and wellbeing and adversely affect their mental state. Obesity which is present in more than 50% of PCOS women results in high degree of dissatisfaction with the physical appearance. The infertility concern also exerts emotional distress to PCOS women and this leads to a loss of womanhood and motherhood leaving them long term depressed and anxious. Thus, challenges to female identity and self-image due to acne, hirsutism, obesity, infertility and long-lasting health risk impair the quality of living and potentially affect the mental and emotional wellbeing. A plethora of studies have shown that PCOS women are more likely to suffer from psychiatric disorders like depression, anxiety, eating disorders, drug-related behavior and psychosexual dysfunction compared to female controls. Recent systematic review and meta-analysis also reveals that PCOS women are more than five times, more likely to have moderate to extreme symptoms of anxiety and more than three times, more likely to have symptoms of depression and further suggests that PCOS is a deeply stigmatizing condition [59]. Several studies have found an association between PCOS women and decreased health related quality of life [60, 61]. The other important element of psychosocial effect in PCOS is the detrimental influence of mood disturbance, poor self-esteem and decreased psychological well-being on motivation and ability to achieve and maintain effective lifestyle improvements that are important to this disorder. Effective screening and appropriate management of all psychiatric co-morbidities are important for the quality care of affected individuals and will enhance well-being and compliance to lifestyles and medical treatments.

Pregnancy Complications

PCOS women are at greater risk of pregnancy and delivery complications. Several meta-analyses have assessed the relationship of pregnancy and delivery complications in PCOS women and demonstrated an increase in the risk for Gestational Diabetes Mellitus (GDM), pregnancy induced hypertension, pre-eclampsia, miscarriage and caesarean section in these women compared to women without PCOS, all of which will independently contribute to adverse neonatal complications [62-66]. However, data concerning the adverse fetal outcomes in PCOS women is ambiguous. Considering the complexity of the syndrome and confounding factors related with pregnancy complications, various risk factors can contribute to the high rate of pregnancy complications in PCOS women. The basic diagnostic features of PCOS, variations in the hormonal and metabolic parameters between different phenotypes of PCOS would strongly affect the observed obstetric and neonatal outcomes either independently or in concert. Further, majority of PCOS patients present with anovulatory infertility which can also play an independent role in pregnancy complications in these women. The meta-analysis which included 63 studies reported that the association of PCOS with pregnancy complications varied with PCOS phenotypes, geographic continent and quality of study. The association of PCOS with these outcomes worsens with hyperandrogenic phenotype, particular regional continents, in high quality research, but declines in assisted pregnancy [67]. However, recent meta-analysis has reported PCOS as an independent risk for experiencing increased risk of pre-term birth, caesarean section, Pre-labor Rupture of Membranes (PPROM), placental abruption and post-partum maternal infections after addressing all the potential confounders [68]. Another recent meta-analysis has reported higher rate of GDM and more than double, increased risk of pregnancy induced hypertension and pre-eclampsia in PCOS women, which after stratification of confounding factors like age and BMI remained significant [62]. It is also reported that infants born to mothers with PCOS are almost four times smaller in gestational age and are considered to be at higher risk for developing metabolic aberrations like obesity, early insulin resistance and even PCOS in the girl child [69]. Taken into account the increased prevalence of overweight/obesity in PCOS women plus the significantly increased body weight during gestation period of PCOS women compared to healthy controls, it further adversely affects the prevalence of pre-term birth or birth weight of the PCOS newborn child and is also associated with increased odds of childhood obesity. Therefore, expecting PCOS women must be informed of the associated risks of pregnancy in order to strengthen the close maternal and neonatal surveillance and as a result of which early preventive management strategies can be performed especially for the high-risk groups with severe phenotypes.

Cancer

Regarding the long term risk, studies have also focused on the risk of several cancers in PCOS women. It is suggested that PCOS women are at increased risk of endometrial cancer. The factors known to increase the risk of endometrial cancer include obesity, long term unopposed estrogen use, infertility, hypertension and diabetes and many of these manifestations are associated with PCOS. The pathways shared by these two conditions have not been thoroughly explored, and most studies that focused on the association between endometrial cancer and PCOS are based on the assumption that prolonged anovulation is the significant cause in both conditions. Chronic anovulation results in elevated estrogen levels and affects the endometrium [70, 71]. Evidences also suggest the association between PCOS and increased ovarian cancer risk. The factors that increase the risk of ovarian cancer include family history of ovarian cancer, age, infertility treatment and aided fertilization, obesity and menopausal hormone replacement [72]. In PCOS menstrual irregularity, increased ovarian androgen secretion and anovulation appears to increase the chance of developing epithelial ovarian cancer owing to abnormal hormonal environment. There have only been few studies highlighting the possible association between PCOS and ovarian cancer with inconsistent reports. Infertility by itself is suggested by studies to increase the risk of borderline and aggressive ovarian tumors [73, 74]. Further, the possible association between breast cancer and PCOS has been explored over the last two decades due to similarities between the breast cancer risk factors and clinical features of PCOS which include obesity, hyperandrogenemia and hyperinsulinemia. However, the findings of studies that examined the relation between breast cancer and PCOS remain contradictory. Some studies reported increased risk of breast cancer in PCOS women and some studies reported no significant increase in the risk of breast cancer in PCOS women [75, 76].

PCOS Pathogenesis Aspects

The pathogenesis of PCOS is not well understood and remains an open question. It is thought to be complex and multifaceted and involves the interplay between genetic, epigenetic and environmental elements that contribute interdependently to its broad range of clinical picture as shown in Figure 3. Over the years several theories have been suggested to describe the pathogenesis of PCOS. The following are the main pathophysiological theories for PCOS.

Ovarian and Adrenal Hyperandrogenism

Hyperandrogenism observed in approximately 85% of PCOS women represents the main clinical presentation of PCOS and is considered to result from the dysfunctional secretion of ovarian and adrenal androgens [14]. Under normal scenario, ovaries and adrenal glands contribute nearly equal to the production of androgens and its precursors in response to their corresponding topical hormones luteinizing hormone (LH) and Adrenocorticotropic hormone (ACTH).

Cholesterol is the precursor for all steroid hormones with cell of ovary and each zones of adrenal gland expressing specific enzymes essential for suitable steroid production as described in figure 4. Briefly ovarian theca cells under the influence of LH produce testosterone and androstenedione which are taken up by the ovarian granulosa cells where the enzyme P450aromatase under the influence of FSH converts them into estradiol. Nearly half of testosterone arises from its direct secretion by the ovaries and adrenal glands, while the other half originates from the peripheral conversion of circulating androstenedione, which in itself results from relatively equivalent ovarian and adrenal secretion. In PCOS, ovaries contribute up to 60% of the androgens and remaining 40% is produced by adrenals [77].

Ovarian hyperandrogenism is attributed to inherent steroidogenic impairment of theca cells. In vitro and clinical PCOS studies of theca cells have demonstrated an increase in androgen biosynthesis and increased expression levels of various steroidogenic enzymes which includes cytochrome P450 cholesterol side chain cleavage enzyme (CYP11A1), 17α-hydroxylase/17–20 lyase (CYP17α1) and 3β-hydroxysteroid dehydrogenase (HSD3B2) [78, 79].

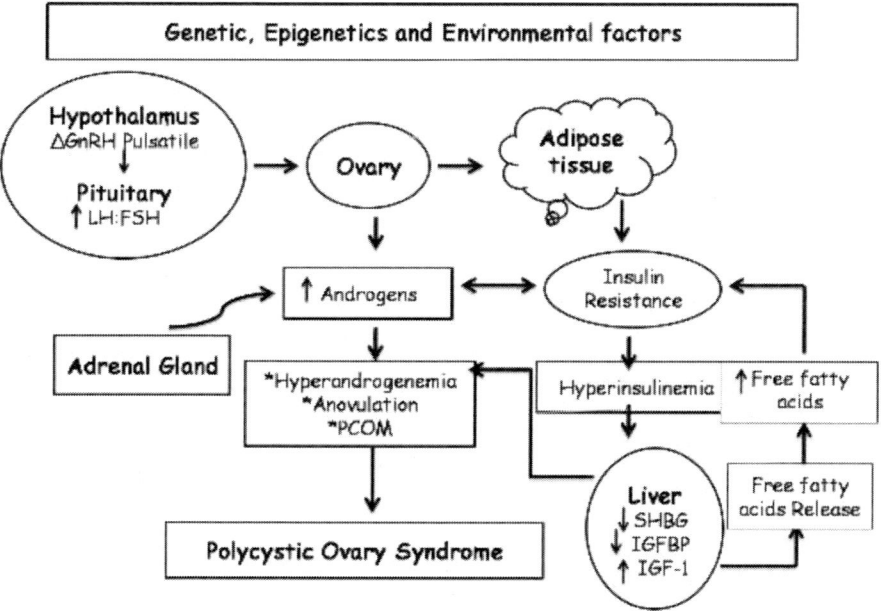

Figure 3. Pathogenesis of Polycystic Ovary Syndrome (PCOS).

These three enzymes function at different stages of the pathway of androgen synthesis as seen in figure 4. Increased insulin and LH levels seem to intensify the underlying abnormality of steroidogenesis [80]. In addition, many of the follicles in PCOS ovaries have been demonstrated to have hypertrophy of theca interna i.e., increased proliferation of theca cells, resulting in increased number of differentiated steroidogenic cells than normal in non PCOS cells. Impaired function of granulosa cell also appears to result in hyperandrogenism in PCOS. In normal PCOS ovaries granulosa cells convert greater part of androstenedione produced by theca cells into estrone and subsequently to estradiol [81]. It is reported that small antral follicles in polycystic ovarian biopsies express low levels of estradiol and reduced mRNA aromatase expression compared with non PCOS dominant follicles. Intrafollicular levels of androgens appear to increase in antral follicles suggesting the lack of sufficient aromatase activity and hence reduced conversion of androgens into estrogen [82]. Also, it is demonstrated that PCOS ovaries express increased activity of 5α-reductase and thousand-fold greater androstenedione follicular fluid levels, a competitive inhibitor of aromatase activity which results in failure to develop dominant follicles. The transition to dominant follicle is characterized by increased expression of aromatase and reduced activity of 5α-reductase to almost undetectable levels [83].

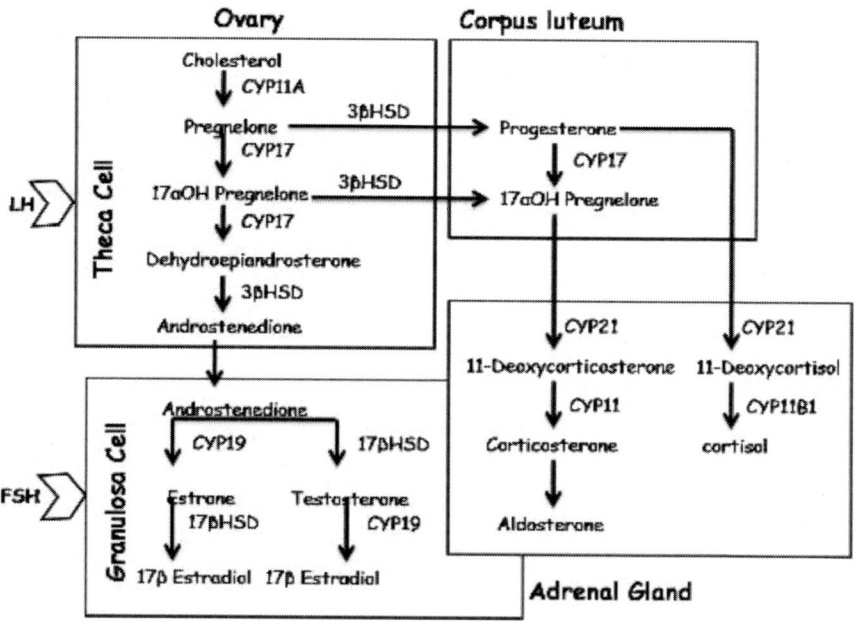

Figure 4. Overview of steroidogenesis.

As a whole, the above defects are likely to result in decreased activity of aromatase enzyme, androstenedione and failure to achieve dominant follicles. A significant number of PCOS patients also present with adrenal androgen excess demonstrated by increased levels of dehydroepiandrosterone sulfate (DHEAS). PCOS patients have reported a systematic hypersecretion of adrenocortical products in response to stimulation by ACTH, mainly attributed to hyperresponsivity of adrenal androgens to stimulation of ACTH and enhanced activity of $\Delta^5 17$-OH. The mechanisms behind these anomalies remain unknown. However, it has been suggested that variety of factors including increased ovarian steroids, altered cortical metabolism, hyperinsulinemia and factors regulating glucose disposal can play a role [84].

Alterations in Gonadotropins

PCOS women demonstrate a deregulation of GnRH pulse generator activities, with a highly disproportionate secretion of LH, relatively decreased secretion of FSH and an increased LH/FSH ratio [85, 86]. The reproductive system is regulated by the HPG (Hypothalamic-pituitary-gonadal axis) in which the release of LH and FSH from the anterior pituitary gonadotrophs is triggered by the pulsatile release of GnRH from the hypothalamus and controls follicular dynamics, ovulation and ovarian steroidogenesis. LH acts predominantly on the ovary theca cells carrying LH receptors and stimulates the release of androgens. FSH on the other hand acts on granulosa cells of the ovary and the converts the androgens produced in the theca cells into estrogens, primarily estradiol, which is important for the formation of follicles. It is therefore reasonable to conclude that the altered secretory profiles of gonadotropin may have an effect on the characteristic features of PCOS which includes ovarian dysfunction and hyperandrogenism. Hyperandrogenemia, in turn, causes a decline in feedback sensitivity of both progesterone and estrogen in gonadotropin hypothalamic cells, promoting hypersecretion of GnRH and LH and therefore representing the first of many pathophysiological cycles in which hyperandrogenism plays a critical role in the development and progression of PCOS, while at the same time ensuring the existence of clinical presentation of hyperandrogenism [81].

Insulin Resistance

Insulin resistance and compensatory hyperinsulinemia is considered to play a vital role in PCOS pathogenesis and responsible for many of its phenotypic characteristics. A number of mechanisms have been suggested in PCOS for the development of insulin resistance. The primary one involves the post binding defects in insulin signaling owing to increased serine phosphorylation and reduced tyrosine phosphorylation of insulin receptor and insulin receptor substrate-1, which influences metabolic pathways in both classical pathways (skeletal muscles and adipocytes) and ovaries [87]. Reduced abundance of insulin receptor-β in omental adipose tissue, reduced GLUT4 (Glucose Transporter 4) in subcutaneous adipocytes contributing to reduced uptake of glucose, mitochondrial dysfunction, constitutive serine kinase activation in MAPK-ERK (Mitogen-Activated Protein Kinase/ Extracellular Signal-Regulated Kinases) pathway and genetic perturbation of insulin signaling in central nervous system are additional factors which contribute to the development of insulin resistance in PCOS [87]. In PCOS the central paradox is that insulin acts via its cognate receptor and promotes ovarian steroidogenesis amid insulin resistance towards glucose metabolism. This paradox can be attributed to the presence of systemic defect disrupting the metabolic and not the mitogenic activity of insulin as observed in skin fibroblast of PCOS [88, 89]. Insulin acts directly on the ovaries and increase the androgen production by stimulating a bifunctional enzyme cytochrome P450c17α [90, 91]. Insulin also acts synergistically with LH on the ovarian theca cells and stimulates the production of androgens [92, 93]. Another adverse effect of hyperinsulinemia on the ovaries of women with PCOS involves arresting the growth of ovarian follicles up to a size of 5 to 10 mm and preventing ovulation [94, 95]. Insulin also acts as co-gonadotropin that enhances the LH activity by stimulating the insulin and IGF ovarian receptors or indirectly intensifying the sensitivity to GnRH stimulation by increasing the amplitude of LH serum pulse. Insulin can also increase ovarian androgen production by reducing the production of sex hormone binding globulin (SHBG) in liver, thereby increasing the bioavailable androgen levels [96]. Hyperinsulinemia further alleviates the PCOS pathogenesis by reducing the production of insulin like growth factor-1 binding proteins (IGFBP) in liver and ovary, resulting in increased IGF-I availability, which in turn improves insulin activity both in the liver (further resulting in reduced SHBG levels) and ovaries; increases the ovarian IGF type 1 receptors and thus amplifies IGF-I and IGF-II ovarian action and accelerates the amplitude of GnRH stimulated LH pulse; resulting in PCOS characteristic features- hyperandrogenemia, oligo/anovulation, production of multiple cystic follicles in the ovaries and follicular atrophy [97]. Androgens in turn can lead back to insulin resistance by increasing the free fatty acid levels and by changing the structure and functionality of muscle tissues, perpetuating a vicious cycle of insulin resistance-hyperinsulinemia-hyperandrogenemia.

Role of Genetic, Environmental and Epigenetic Factors

Genetic factors are also known to play a key role in the development of this syndrome. Family-based research, twin studies, GWAS (Genome-Wide Association Studies) and fetal programming studies suggest that there is indeed a significant hereditary element to the condition [98]. Distinct genetic pathways, which include autosomal dominant, modified autosomal dominant, X-linked dominant and other multifactorial have been suggested, but still the exact mode of inheritance of PCOS has not yet been identified [99]. Numerous candidate genes are being suggested to contribute to pathogenicity. Well not only the genetic variants in steroid hormone biosynthetic pathways have been documented but also genes related to gonadotropin secretion and action, insulin secretion and action, energy homeostasis and inflammation among others have been studied which are the characteristic features of PCOS [100]. Besides that, environmental factors including diet and nutrition, environmental toxins, a socioeconomic status, and geography are involved in etiology, prevalence and are believed to affect the phenotype of PCOS [101]. Environmental insults, beginning from early life and continuing throughout the life span can affect susceptible women who eventually show the clinical phenotype of PCOS. Diet is emerging as the main environmental determinant of PCOS. Over nutrition contributing to obesity is generally accepted as having an aggravating effect [102]. Lifestyle also has a significant influence on the clinical manifestations of PCOS. Gaining weight deteriorates the reproductive and metabolic aberrations of PCOS, as demonstrated by increased degree of obesity, menstrual irregularity, hyperandrogenism, insulin resistance in PCOS women with more intense phenotypes. Sedentary lifestyle alone as well leads to metabolic dysfunctions in women with PCOS, since physical activities without losing weight lowers body adipose tissue and improves insulin resistance [36]. There is mountain of evidence that environmental toxins have an important effect on human wellbeing and reproductive health. Environmental toxins are described as chemical substances in the environment that have detrimental effects on organic species. Environmental exposure to industrial products like Bisphenol A has been shown to act as endocrine disruptor in the pathogenesis of PCOS and may exacerbate its clinical course [103].

Environmental factors may also play a crucial role in early stages of human development. Studies from animal models demonstrate that exposure to maternal hyperandrogenism at crucial period of fetal development may induce permanent changes in the physiology of fetus that may contribute to the development of PCOS later in life. Clinical studies to evaluate implications of maternal androgens in fetus are not possible in humans. However, studies were conducted on humans to affirm the significance of this theory. Examples of female prenatal androgenized fetuses are those having congenital adrenal hyperplasia due to the deficiency of 21-hydroxylase or congenital virilizing tumor. Even after normalization of hyperandrogenemia with post-natal therapies or tumor removal, these women exhibit PCOS characteristics [104, 105]. Likewise, female fetuses of women with rare conditions like abnormalities in the gene of sex hormone-binding globulin and p-450 aromatase gene are reported to develop characteristics of PCOS later in life [106, 107]. The potential role of PCOS on its own as a source of excess prenatal androgens was evaluated in a study in which maternal androgen level is reported to be significantly elevated in pregnant PCOS women compared to healthy pregnant women [108]. It is believed that prenatal androgen exposure to the offspring of PCOS women may result in the development of PCOS in adulthood. PCOS women are also reported to have increased insulin resistance during pregnancy which has been found to be linked with adverse pregnancy complications like preeclampsia, gestational diabetes and preterm labor [109, 110]. The male child of PCOS women has been found to have increased prevalence of dyslipidemia, insulin resistance and type 2 diabetes in adult life [111]. There may also be present developmental delay in fetus of PCOS mother which could be related to increased testosterone and insulin resistance [112]. Also, PCOS women may deliver the infants at small gestation age with higher prevalence compared to control women [113]. Apart from the above discussed associations increased prenatal androgen exposure is also believed to result in low birth weight during the intrauterine period. Low birth weight in girls has been shown in studies to be associated with the development of early pubarche preceded by insulin resistance and compensatory hyperinsulinemia, hyperandrogenism and dyslipidemia during adolescence. It has been suggested that there may be an early common origin for such characteristics [114, 115]. Low birth weight indicating intrauterine nutritional insufficiency is reported by various studies to be linked with an increased incidence of developing characteristics of metabolic syndrome like insulin resistance, obesity, hypertension and type 2 diabetes [116]. The development of insulin resistance is thought to be closely linked to the body anticipating the presence of undernourishment for developing fetus. Any such fetus or infant will have stunted growth and is prone to develop PCOS later in life when exposed to excess nutrition. These associations appear to be the result of programming by which stimuli or insult during an early sensitive period of life may lead to considerable alterations in metabolism and physiology and hence lead to the hypothesis of fetal origin of adult diseases [116, 117].

Recently, the role of epigenetic factors has been studied in the PCOS pathogenesis. Particular emphasis has been shown in the role of micro-RNAs (miRNAs) which are the epigenetic regulators that would bridge the genetic and epigenetic roots of this condition. miRNAs are small, endogenous, non-coding, single stranded, RNA sequences of 21-25 nucleotides that negatively regulate the gene expression at post transcription level, by binding in a sequence specific manner to messenger RNAs [118]. The presence of regulatory feedback mechanisms between miRNAs, their regulatory targets and proteins allows for the inhibition and enhancement of a particular signal. As a consequence, changes in the expression patterns of small fraction of miRNAs can lead to many diseases. Moreover, miRNAs circulate freely in the blood and assessment of circulatory miRNAs has the benefit of easy recognition, stability and being degradation proof and therefore has the potential to be signatory markers of the diseases [119]. Altered expression pattern of miRNAs has been associated with several diseases including diabetes, nonalcoholic fatty liver disease, cancer and recently PCOS [120, 121]. miRNA expression has been documented in PCOS woman's follicular fluid, tissue and circulation and has been shown to be elevated in PCOS women relative to controls with the implication that they have a chance to act as predominant signatory markers and new therapeutic targets in PCOS [121, 122].

Conclusion

In conclusion, PCOS has become the most prevalent disorder of reproductive age women and PCOS phenotype emerges as a longtime challenging issue for the affected women due to its wide range of clinical manifestations like hyperandrogenism, ovulatory dysfunction, polycystic ovaries, infertility, complicated pregnancies and other female reproductive system issues. These females have deranged markers for metabolic syndrome owing to their insulin resistant states and this puts them at higher risk of cardiovascular diseases (CVD), diabetes mellitus, and gynecological cancers among others. The overall quality of life of these women is therefore compromised and adversely influences mood and psychological well-being which is a social issue as whole. Hence, consideration of both physical and mental health of affected individuals is vitally important as part of individualized intervention approach intended to improve the overall clinical outcomes. Further, PCOS remains a complex pathophysiological disorder with no single criteria appropriate for diagnosis and there is still considerable debate on the issue. This problem is aggravated by its high level of heterogeneity and is further complicated by associated endocrine, environmental, genetic and epigenetic factors. In that context continuous research is needed to identify biomarkers that can help in diagnosis, prevention and development of newer therapeutic options regarding the disease.

REFERENCES

[1] Azziz, Ricardo. "Polycystic ovary syndrome." *Obstetrics & Gynecology* 132, no. 2 (2018): 321-336.

[2] Stein, Irving F. "Amenorrhea associated with bilateral polycystic ovaries." *Am J Obstet Gynecol* 29 (1935): 181-191.

[3] Insler, V., and B. Lunenfeld. "Polycystic ovarian disease: a challenge and controversy." *Gynecological Endocrinology* 4, no. 1 (1990): 51-70.

[4] Zawadski, J., and A. Dunaif. *Polycystic ovary syndrome: diagnostic criteria for polycystic ovarian syndrome: towards a rational approach.* (1992): 377-84.

[5] ESHRE, The Rotterdam, and ASRM-Sponsored PCOS Consensus Workshop Group. "Revised 2003 consensus on diagnostic criteria and long-term health risks related to polycystic ovary syndrome." *Fertility and sterility* 81, no. 1 (2004): 19-25.

[6] Azziz, R., E. Carmina, D. Dewailly, E. Diamanti-Kandarakis, H. F. Escobar-Morreale, W. Futterweit, O. E. Janssen et al. "Androgen Excess Society. Positions statement: criteria for defining polycystic ovary syndrome as a predominantly hyperandrogenic syndrome: an Androgen Excess Society guideline." *J Clin Endocrinol Metab* 91, no. 11 (2006): 4237-4245.

[7] Fauser, Bart CJM, Basil C. Tarlatzis, Robert W. Rebar, Richard S. Legro, Adam H. Balen, Roger Lobo, Enrico Carmina et al. "Consensus on women's health aspects of polycystic ovary syndrome (PCOS): the Amsterdam ESHRE/ASRM-Sponsored 3rd PCOS Consensus Workshop Group." *Fertility and sterility* 97, no. 1 (2012): 28-38.

[8] Bozdag, Gurkan, Sezcan Mumusoglu, Dila Zengin, Erdem Karabulut, and Bulent Okan Yildiz. "The prevalence and phenotypic features of

polycystic ovary syndrome: a systematic review and meta-analysis." *Human Reproduction* 31, no. 12 (2016): 2841-2855.

[9] Nidhi, Ram, Venkatram Padmalatha, Raghuram Nagarathna, and Ram Amritanshu. "Prevalence of polycystic ovarian syndrome in Indian adolescents." *Journal of pediatric and adolescent gynecology* 24, no. 4 (2011): 223-227.

[10] Nair, M. K. C., Princly Pappachan, Sheila Balakrishnan, M. L. Leena, Babu George, and Paul S. Russell. "Menstrual irregularity and poly cystic ovarian syndrome among adolescent girls—a 2 year follow-up study." *The Indian Journal of Pediatrics* 79, no. 1 (2012): 69-73.

[11] Joshi, Beena, Srabani Mukherjee, Anushree Patil, Ameya Purandare, Sanjay Chauhan, and Rama Vaidya. "A cross-sectional study of polycystic ovarian syndrome among adolescent and young girls in Mumbai, India." *Indian journal of endocrinology and metabolism* 18, no. 3 (2014): 317.

[12] Ganie, Mohd Ashraf, Aafia Rashid, Danendra Sahu, Sobia Nisar, Ishfaq A. Wani, and Junaida Khan. "Prevalence of polycystic ovary syndrome (PCOS) among reproductive age women from Kashmir valley: A cross-sectional study." *International Journal of Gynecology & Obstetrics* 149, no. 2 (2020): 231-236.

[13] Meek, Claire L., Vassiliki Bravis, Abigail Don, and Felicity Kaplan. "Polycystic ovary syndrome and the differential diagnosis of hyperandrogenism." *The Obstetrician & Gynaecologist* 15, no. 3 (2013): 171-176.

[14] Azziz, Ricardo, L. A. Sanchez, E. S. Knochenhauer, C. Moran, J. Lazenby, K. C. Stephens, K. Taylor, and L. R. Boots. "Androgen excess in women: experience with over 1000 consecutive patients." *The Journal of Clinical Endocrinology & Metabolism* 89, no. 2 (2004): 453-462.

[15] Patel, Seema. "Polycystic ovary syndrome (PCOS), an inflammatory, systemic, lifestyle endocrinopathy." *The Journal of steroid biochemistry and molecular biology* 182 (2018): 27-36.

[16] Gainder, Shalini, and Bharti Sharma. "Update on management of polycystic ovarian syndrome for dermatologists." *Indian dermatology online journal* 10, no. 2 (2019): 97.

[17] Espinós, Juan J., Joaquim Calaf, Josep Estadella, and Miguel A. Checa. "Hirsutism scoring in polycystic ovary syndrome: concordance between clinicians' and patients' self-scoring." *Fertility and sterility* 94, no. 7 (2010): 2815-2816.

[18] Witchel, Selma Feldman, Sharon E. Oberfield, and Alexia S. Peña. "Polycystic ovary syndrome: pathophysiology, presentation, and treatment with emphasis on adolescent girls." *Journal of the Endocrine Society* 3, no. 8 (2019): 1545-1573.

[19] Keen, Mohammad Abid, Iffat Hassan Shah, and Gousia Sheikh. "Cutaneous manifestations of polycystic ovary syndrome: A cross-sectional clinical study." *Indian dermatology online journal* 8, no. 2 (2017): 104.

[20] Makrantonaki, Evgenia, Ruta Ganceviciene, and Christos C. Zouboulis. "An update on the role of the sebaceous gland in the pathogenesis of acne." *Dermato-endocrinology* 3, no. 1 (2011): 41-49.

[21] WD, II James. "Clinical practice. Acne." *N Engl J Med* 352 (2005): 1463-1472.

[22] Dalgard, F., Åke Svensson, J. Ø. Holm, and J. Sundby. "Self-reported skin morbidity in Oslo. Associations with sociodemographic factors among adults in a cross-sectional study." *British journal of dermatology* 151, no. 2 (2004): 452-457.

[23] Galobardes, B., G. Davey Smith, M. Jeffreys, and P. McCarron. "Has acne increased? Prevalence of acne history among university students between 1948 and 1968. The Glasgow Alumni Cohort Study." *British Journal of Dermatology* 152, no. 4 (2005): 824-825.

[24] Gollnick, Harald P., and Christos C. Zouboulis. "Not all acne is acne vulgaris." *Deutsches Ärzteblatt International* 111, no. 17 (2014): 301.

[25] Ebede, Tobechi L., Emily L. Arch, and Diane Berson. "Hormonal treatment of acne in women." *The Journal of clinical and aesthetic dermatology* 2, no. 12 (2009): 16.

[26] Gebauer, Kurt. "Acne in adolescents." *Australian family physician* 46, no. 12 (2017): 892-895.

[27] Zaenglein, Andrea L., Arun L. Pathy, Bethanee J. Schlosser, Ali Alikhan, Hilary E. Baldwin, Diane S. Berson, Whitney P. Bowe et al. "Guidelines of care for the management of acne vulgaris." *Journal of the American Academy of Dermatology* 74, no. 5 (2016): 945-973.

[28] Sirmans, Susan M., and Kristen A. Pate. "Epidemiology, diagnosis, and management of polycystic ovary syndrome." *Clinical epidemiology* 6 (2014): 1.

[29] Borgia, Francesco, Salvatore Cannavò, Fabrizio Guarneri, Serafinella Patrizia Cannavò, Mario Vaccaro, and Biagio Guarneri. "Correlation between endocrinological parameters and acne severity in adult women." *Acta Dermatovenereologica-Stockholm-* 84, no. 3 (2004): 201-204.

[30] Slayden, Scott M., Carlos Moran, W. Mitchell Sams Jr, Larry R. Boots, and Ricardo Azziz. "Hyperandrogenemia in patients presenting with acne." *Fertility and sterility* 75, no. 5 (2001): 889-892.

[31] Ramos, Paulo Müller, and Hélio Amante Miot. "Female pattern hair loss: a clinical and pathophysiological review." *Anais brasileiros de dermatologia* 90, no. 4 (2015): 529-543.

[32] Ludwig, Erich. "Classification of the types of androgenetic alopecia (common baldness) occurring in the female sex." *British Journal of Dermatology* 97, no. 3 (1977): 247-254.

[33] Melo, Anderson Sanches, Rui Alberto Ferriani, and Paula Andrea Navarro. "Treatment of infertility in women with polycystic ovary syndrome: approach to clinical practice." *Clinics* 70, no. 11 (2015): 765-769.

[34] Dewailly, Didier, Marla E. Lujan, Enrico Carmina, Marcelle I. Cedars, Joop Laven, Robert J. Norman, and Héctor F. Escobar-Morreale. "Definition and significance of polycystic ovarian morphology: a task force report from the Androgen Excess and Polycystic Ovary Syndrome Society." *Human reproduction update* 20, no. 3 (2014): 334-352.

[35] Ng, Marie, Tom Fleming, Margaret Robinson, Blake Thomson, Nicholas Graetz, Christopher Margono, Erin C. Mullany et al. "Global, regional, and national prevalence of overweight and obesity in children and adults during 1980–2013: a systematic analysis for the Global Burden of Disease Study 2013." *The Lancet* 384, no. 9945 (2014): 766-781.

[36] Barber, Thomas M., Petra Hanson, Martin O. Weickert, and Stephen Franks. "Obesity and polycystic ovary syndrome: implications for pathogenesis and novel management strategies." *Clinical Medicine Insights: Reproductive Health* 13 (2019): 1179558119874042.

[37] Lim, S. S., Robert J. Norman, M. J. Davies, and L. J. Moran. "The effect of obesity on polycystic ovary syndrome: a systematic review and meta-analysis." *Obesity Reviews* 14, no. 2 (2013): 95-109.

[38] Alvarez-Blasco, Francisco, José I. Botella-Carretero, José L. San Millán, and Héctor F. Escobar-Morreale. "Prevalence and characteristics of the polycystic ovary syndrome in overweight and obese women." *Archives of internal medicine* 166, no. 19 (2006): 2081-2086.

[39] Dunaif, Andrea, and Carol Beth Book. "Insulin resistance in the polycystic ovary syndrome." *Clinical research in diabetes and obesity* (1997): 249-274.

[40] Dunaif, Andrea, Karen R. Segal, Walter Futterweit, and Areta Dobrjansky. "Profound peripheral insulin resistance, independent of obesity, in polycystic ovary syndrome." *Diabetes* 38, no. 9 (1989): 1165-1174.

[41] Barthelmess, Erin K., and Rajesh K. Naz. "Polycystic ovary syndrome: current status and future perspective." *Frontiers in bioscience (Elite edition)* 6 (2014): 104.

[42] Moran, Lisa J., Marie L. Misso, Robert A. Wild, and Robert J. Norman. "Impaired glucose tolerance, type 2 diabetes and metabolic syndrome in polycystic ovary syndrome: a systematic review and meta-analysis." *Human reproduction update* 16, no. 4 (2010): 347-363.

[43] Rosenfield, Robert L., and David A. Ehrmann. "The pathogenesis of polycystic ovary syndrome (PCOS): the hypothesis of PCOS as functional ovarian hyperandrogenism revisited." *Endocrine reviews* 37, no. 5 (2016): 467-520.

[44] Diamanti-Kandarakis, Evanthia, and Andrea Dunaif. "Insulin resistance and the polycystic ovary syndrome revisited: an update on mechanisms and implications." *Endocrine reviews* 33, no. 6 (2012): 981-1030.

[45] Phiske, Meghana Madhukar. "An approach to acanthosis nigricans." *Indian dermatology online journal* 5, no. 3 (2014): 239.

[46] O'Brien, Brooke, Rachana Dahiya, and Rebecca Kimble. "Hyperandrogenism, insulin resistance and acanthosis nigricans (HAIR-AN syndrome): an extreme subphenotype of polycystic ovary syndrome." *BMJ Case Reports CP* 13, no. 4 (2020): e231749.

[47] Kim, Jin Ju, and Young Min Choi. "Dyslipidemia in women with polycystic ovary syndrome." *Obstetrics & gynecology science* 56, no. 3 (2013): 137.

[48] Wild, Robert A., P. C. Painter, Patricia B. Coulson, Kayla B. Carruth, and G. B. Ranney. "Lipoprotein lipid concentrations and cardiovascular risk in women with polycystic ovary syndrome." *The Journal of Clinical Endocrinology & Metabolism* 61, no. 5 (1985): 946-951.

[49] Wild, Robert A., and Mary J. Bartholomew. "The influence of body weight on lipoprotein lipids in patients with polycystic ovary syndrome." *American journal of obstetrics and gynecology* 159, no. 2 (1988): 423-427.

[50] Liu, Qi, Yuan-jie Xie, Li-hua Qu, Meng-xia Zhang, and Zhong-cheng Mo. "Dyslipidemia involvement in the development of polycystic ovary syndrome." *Taiwanese Journal of Obstetrics and Gynecology* 58, no. 4 (2019): 447-453.

[51] Kakoly, N. S., M. B. Khomami, A. E. Joham, S. D. Cooray, M. L. Misso, R. J. Norman, C. L. Harrison, S. Ranasinha, H. J. Teede, and L. J. Moran. "Ethnicity, obesity and the prevalence of impaired glucose tolerance and type 2 diabetes in PCOS: a systematic review

and meta-regression." *Human Reproduction Update* 24, no. 4 (2018): 455-467.
[52] Gambineri, Alessandra, Laura Patton, Paola Altieri, Uberto Pagotto, Carmine Pizzi, Lamberto Manzoli, and Renato Pasquali. "Polycystic ovary syndrome is a risk factor for type 2 diabetes: results from a long-term prospective study." *Diabetes* 61, no. 9 (2012): 2369-2374.
[53] Salley, Kelsey ES, Edmond P. Wickham, Kai I. Cheang, Paulina A. Essah, Nicole W. Karjane, and John E. Nestler. "Position statement: glucose intolerance in polycystic ovary syndrome—a position statement of the Androgen Excess Society." *The Journal of Clinical Endocrinology & Metabolism* 92, no. 12 (2007): 4546-4556.
[54] Celik, Cem, Nicel Tasdemir, Remzi Abali, Ercan Bastu, and Murat Yilmaz. "Progression to impaired glucose tolerance or type 2 diabetes mellitus in polycystic ovary syndrome: a controlled follow-up study." *Fertility and sterility* 101, no. 4 (2014): 1123-1128.
[55] Teede, Helena, Amanda Deeks, and Lisa Moran. "Polycystic ovary syndrome: a complex conditions with psychological, reproductive and metabolic manifestations that impact on health across the lifespan." *BMC medicine* 8, no. 1 (2010): 1-10.
[56] Scicchitano, Pietro, Ilaria Dentamaro, Rosa Carbonara, Gabriella Bulzis, Annamaria Dachille, Paola Caputo, Roberta Riccardi, Manuela Locorotondo, Cosimo Mandurino, and Marco Matteo Ciccone. "Cardiovascular risk in women with PCOS." *International journal of endocrinology and metabolism* 10, no. 4 (2012): 611.
[57] Osibogun, Olatokunbo, Oluseye Ogunmoroti, and Erin D. Michos. "Polycystic ovary syndrome and cardiometabolic risk: opportunities for cardiovascular disease prevention." *Trends in cardiovascular medicine* (2019).
[58] Studen, Katica Bajuk, and Marija Pfeifer. "Cardiometabolic risk in polycystic ovary syndrome." *Endocrine connections* 7, no. 7 (2018): R238-R251.
[59] Yin, Xican, Yinan Ji, Cecilia Lai Wan Chan, and Celia Hoi Yan Chan. "The mental health of women with polycystic ovary syndrome: a

systematic review and meta-analysis." *Archives of Women's Mental Health* (2020): 1-17

[60] Cooney, Laura G., Iris Lee, Mary D. Sammel, and Anuja Dokras. "High prevalence of moderate and severe depressive and anxiety symptoms in polycystic ovary syndrome: a systematic review and meta-analysis." *Human Reproduction* 32, no. 5 (2017): 1075-1091.

[61] Brutocao, Claire, Feras Zaiem, Mouaz Alsawas, Allison S. Morrow, M. Hassan Murad, and Asma Javed. "Psychiatric disorders in women with polycystic ovary syndrome: a systematic review and meta-analysis." *Endocrine* 62, no. 2 (2018): 318-325.

[62] Yu, Hai-Feng, Hong-Su Chen, Da-Pang Rao, and Jian Gong. "Association between polycystic ovary syndrome and the risk of pregnancy complications: a PRISMA-compliant systematic review and meta-analysis." *Medicine* 95, no. 51 (2016).

[63] Toulis, Konstantinos A., Dimitrios G. Goulis, Efstratios M. Kolibianakis, Christos A. Venetis, Basil C. Tarlatzis, and Ioannis Papadimas. "Risk of gestational diabetes mellitus in women with polycystic ovary syndrome: a systematic review and a meta-analysis." *Fertility and sterility* 92, no. 2 (2009): 667-677.

[64] Qin, Jun Z., Li H. Pang, Mu J. Li, Xiao J. Fan, Ru D. Huang, and Hong Y. Chen. "Obstetric complications in women with polycystic ovary syndrome: a systematic review and meta-analysis." *Reproductive Biology and Endocrinology* 11, no. 1 (2013): 1-14.

[65] Kjerulff, Lucinda E., Luis Sanchez-Ramos, and Daniel Duffy. "Pregnancy outcomes in women with polycystic ovary syndrome: a metaanalysis." *American journal of obstetrics and gynecology* 204, no. 6 (2011): 558-e1.

[66] Boomsma, C. M., M. J. C. Eijkemans, E. G. Hughes, G. H. A. Visser, B. C. J. M. Fauser, and N. S. Macklon. "A meta-analysis of pregnancy outcomes in women with polycystic ovary syndrome." *Human reproduction update* 12, no. 6 (2006): 673-683.

[67] Bahri Khomami, Mahnaz, Anju E. Joham, Jacqueline A. Boyle, Terhi Piltonen, Michael Silagy, Chavy Arora, Marie L. Misso, Helena J. Teede, and Lisa J. Moran. "Increased maternal pregnancy

complications in polycystic ovary syndrome appear to be independent of obesity—A systematic review, meta-analysis, and meta-regression." *Obesity Reviews* 20, no. 5 (2019): 659-674.

[68] Mills, Ginevra, Ahmad Badeghiesh, Eva Suarthana, Haitham Baghlaf, and Michael H. Dahan. "Associations between polycystic ovary syndrome and adverse obstetric and neonatal outcomes: a population study of 9.1 million births." *Human Reproduction* 35, no. 8 (2020): 1914-1921.

[69] de Wilde, Marlieke A., Marije Lamain-de Ruiter, Susanne M. Veltman-Verhulst, Anncke Kwee, Joop S. Laven, Cornelis B. Lambalk, Marinus JC Eijkemans, Arie Franx, Bart CJM Fauser, and Maria PH Koster. "Increased rates of complications in singleton pregnancies of women previously diagnosed with polycystic ovary syndrome predominantly in the hyperandrogenic phenotype." *Fertility and sterility* 108, no. 2 (2017): 333-340.

[70] Gopal, Mira, Stephen Duntley, Matt Uhles, and Hrayr Attarian. "The role of obesity in the increased prevalence of obstructive sleep apnea syndrome in patients with polycystic ovarian syndrome." *Sleep medicine* 3, no. 5 (2002): 401-404.

[71] Robert, A. "Wild. Long-term health consequences of PCOS." *Human reproduction update* 8 (2002): 231-241.

[72] Liu, Zhen, Ting-Ting Zhang, Jing-Jing Zhao, Su-Fen Qi, Pei Du, Dian-Wu Liu, and Qing-Bao Tian. "The association between overweight, obesity and ovarian cancer: a meta-analysis." *Japanese journal of clinical oncology* 45, no. 12 (2015): 1107-1115.

[73] Mosgaard, Berit Jul, Øjvind Lidegaard, Susanne Krüger Kjaer, Geert Schou, and Anders Nyboe Andersen. "Infertility, fertility drugs, and invasive ovarian cancer: a case-control study." *Fertility and sterility* 67, no. 6 (1997): 1005-1012.

[74] Mosgaard, Berit Jul, Øjvind Lidegaard, Susanne Krüger Kjær, Geert Schou, and Anders Nyboe Andersen. "Ovarian stimulation and borderline ovarian tumors: a case-control study." *Fertility and sterility* 70, no. 6 (1998): 1049-1055.

[75] Pierpoint, T., P. M. McKeigue, A. J. Isaacs, S. H. Wild, and H. S. Jacobs. "Mortality of women with polycystic ovary syndrome at long-term follow-up." *Journal of clinical epidemiology* 51, no. 7 (1998): 581-586.

[76] Atiomo, William U., Essam El-Mahdi, and Paul Hardiman. "Familial associations in women with polycystic ovary syndrome." *Fertility and sterility* 80, no. 1 (2003): 143-145.

[77] Cedars, Marcelle I., Kenneth A. Steingold, Dominique de Ziegler, Philip S. Lapolt, R. Jeffrey Chang, and Howard L. Judd. "Long-term administration of gonadotropin-releasing hormone agonist and dexamethasone: assessment of the adrenal role in ovarian dysfunction." *Fertility and Sterility* 57, no. 3 (1992): 495-500.

[78] Nelson, Velen L., Richard S. Legro, Jerome F. Strauss III, and Jan M. McAllister. "Augmented androgen production is a stable steroidogenic phenotype of propagated theca cells from polycystic ovaries." *Molecular endocrinology* 13, no. 6 (1999): 946-957.

[79] Nelson, Velen L., Ke-nan Qin, Robert L. Rosenfield, Jennifer R. Wood, Trevor M. Penning, Richard S. Legro, Jerome F. Strauss III, and Jan M. McAllister. "The biochemical basis for increased testosterone production in theca cells propagated from patients with polycystic ovary syndrome." *The Journal of Clinical Endocrinology & Metabolism* 86, no. 12 (2001): 5925-5933.

[80] Wu, Sheng, Sara Divall, Amanda Nwaopara, Sally Radovick, Fredric Wondisford, CheMyong Ko, and Andrew Wolfe. "Obesity-induced infertility and hyperandrogenism are corrected by deletion of the insulin receptor in the ovarian theca cell." *Diabetes* 63, no. 4 (2014): 1270-1282.

[81] Rosenfield, Robert L., and David A. Ehrmann. "The pathogenesis of polycystic ovary syndrome (PCOS): the hypothesis of PCOS as functional ovarian hyperandrogenism revisited." *Endocrine reviews* 37, no. 5 (2016): 467-520.

[82] Schneyer, Alan L., Toshihiro Fujiwara, Janis Fox, Corrine K. Welt, Judith Adams, Geralyn M. Messerlian, and Ann E. Taylor. "Dynamic changes in the intrafollicular inhibin/activin/follistatin axis during

human follicular development: relationship to circulating hormone concentrations." *The Journal of Clinical Endocrinology & Metabolism* 85, no. 9 (2000): 3319-3330.

[83] Jakimiuk, Artur J., Stacy R. Weitsman, and Denis A. Magoffin. "5α-reductase activity in women with polycystic ovary syndrome." *The Journal of Clinical Endocrinology & Metabolism* 84, no. 7 (1999): 2414-2418.

[84] Yildiz, Bulent O., Enrico Carmina, and Ricardo Azziz. "Hypothalamic-pituitary-adrenal dysfunction in the polycystic ovary syndrome." In *Androgen Excess Disorders in Women*, pp. 213-222. Humana Press, 2006.

[85] Fauser, Bart CJM, Thierry D. Pache, Steven WJ Lamberts, WIM CJ Hop, Frank H. De jong, and Kristine D. Dahl. "Serum bioactive and immunoreactive luteinizing hormone and follicle-stimulating hormone levels in women with cycle abnormalities, with or without polycystic ovarian disease." *The Journal of Clinical Endocrinology & Metabolism* 73, no. 4 (1991): 811-817.

[86] Van Santbrink, Evert Jp, Wim C. Hop, and Bart CJM Fauser. "Classification of normogonadotropic infertility: polycystic ovaries diagnosed by ultrasound versus endocrine characteristics of polycystic ovary syndrome." *Fertility and sterility* 67, no. 3 (1997): 452-458.

[87] Anagnostis, Panagiotis, Basil C. Tarlatzis, and Robert P. Kauffman. "Polycystic ovarian syndrome (PCOS): Long-term metabolic consequences." *Metabolism* 86 (2018): 33-43.

[88] Book, Carol-Beth, and Andrea Dunaif. "Selective insulin resistance in the polycystic ovary syndrome." *The Journal of Clinical Endocrinology & Metabolism* 84, no. 9 (1999): 3110-3116.

[89] Corbould, Anne, Haiyan Zhao, Salida Mirzoeva, Fraser Aird, and Andrea Dunaif. "Enhanced mitogenic signaling in skeletal muscle of women with polycystic ovary syndrome." *Diabetes* 55, no. 3 (2006): 751-759.

[90] Nestler, John E., Daniela J. Jakubowicz, Aida Falcon de Vargas, Carlos Brik, Nitza Quintero, and Francisco Medina. "Insulin

stimulates testosterone biosynthesis by human thecal cells from women with polycystic ovary syndrome by activating its own receptor and using inositolglycan mediators as the signal transduction system." *The Journal of Clinical Endocrinology & Metabolism* 83, no. 6 (1998): 2001-2005.

[91] Conway, Gerard S., Cate Avey, and Gill Rumsby. "Genetics: The tyrosine kinase domain of the insulin receptor gene is normal in women with hyperinsulinaemia and polycystic ovary syndrome." *Human reproduction* 9, no. 9 (1994): 1681-1683.

[92] Cara, José F., and Robert L. Rosenfield. "Insulin-like growth factor I and insulin potentiate luteinizing hormone-induced androgen synthesis by rat ovarian thecal-interstitial cells." *Endocrinology* 123, no. 2 (1988): 733-739.

[93] Hernandez, Eleuterio R., Carol E. Resnick, W. David Holtzclaw, Donna W. PaynE, and Eli y. Adashi. "Insulin as a regulator of androgen biosynthesis by cultured rat ovarian cells: cellular mechanism (s) underlying physiological and pharmacological hormonal actions." *Endocrinology* 122, no. 5 (1988): 2034-2043.

[94] Robinson, S., D. Kiddy, S. V. Gelding, D. Willis, R. Niththyananthan, A. Bush, D. G. Johnston, and S. Franks. "The relationship of insulin insensitivity to menstrual pattern in women with hyperandrogenism and polycystic ovaries." *Clinical endocrinology* 39, no. 3 (1993): 351-355.

[95] Willis, Debbie S., Hazel Watson, Helen D. Mason, Ray Galea, Mark Brincat, and Stephen Franks. "Premature response to luteinizing hormone of granulosa cells from anovulatory women with polycystic ovary syndrome: relevance to mechanism of anovulation." *The Journal of Clinical Endocrinology & Metabolism* 83, no. 11 (1998): 3984-3991.

[96] Cassar, Samantha, Marie L. Misso, William G. Hopkins, Christopher S. Shaw, Helena J. Teede, and Nigel K. Stepto. "Insulin resistance in polycystic ovary syndrome: a systematic review and meta-analysis of euglycaemic–hyperinsulinaemic clamp studies." *Human reproduction* 31, no. 11 (2016): 2619-2631.

[97] Bremer, Andrew A., and Walter L. Miller. "The serine phosphorylation hypothesis of polycystic ovary syndrome: a unifying mechanism for hyperandrogenemia and insulin resistance." *Fertility and sterility* 89, no. 5 (2008): 1039-1048.

[98] Crespo, Raiane P., Tania ASS Bachega, Berenice B. Mendonça, and Larissa G. Gomes. "An update of genetic basis of PCOS pathogenesis." *Archives of endocrinology and metabolism* 62, no. 3 (2018): 352-361.

[99] Franks, Stephen, Neda Gharani, and Mark McCarthy. "Candidate genes in polycystic ovary syndrome." *Human Reproduction Update* 7, no. 4 (2001): 405-410.

[100] Prapas, Nikolaos, A. Karkanaki, Ioannis Prapas, Ioannis Kalogiannidis, I. Katsikis, and D. Panidis. "Genetics of polycystic ovary syndrome." *Hippokratia* 13, no. 4 (2009): 216.

[101] Merkin, Sharon Stein, Jennifer L. Phy, Cynthia K. Sites, and Dongzi Yang. "Environmental determinants of polycystic ovary syndrome." *Fertility and sterility* 106, no. 1 (2016): 16-24.

[102] Diamanti-Kandarakis, Evanthia, Charikleia Christakou, and Evangelos Marinakis. "Phenotypes and enviromental factors: their influence in PCOS." *Current pharmaceutical design* 18, no. 3 (2012): 270-282.

[103] Kawa, Iram Ashaq, Akbar Masood, Mohd Ashraf Ganie, Qudsia Fatima, Humira Jeelani, Saika Manzoor, Syeed Masuma Rizvi, Mohd Muzamil, and Fouzia Rashid. "Bisphenol A (BPA) acts as an endocrine disruptor in women with Polycystic Ovary Syndrome: Hormonal and metabolic evaluation." *Obesity Medicine* 14 (2019): 100090.

[104] Hague, William M., Judith Adams, Christine Rodda, Charles Gd Brook, R. O. S. E. De Bruyn, David B. Grant, and Howard S. Jacobs. "The prevalence of polycystic ovaries in patients with congenital adrenal hyperplasia and their close relatives." *Clinical endocrinology* 33, no. 4 (1990): 501-510.

[105] Barnes, R. B., R. L. Rosenfield, D. A. Ehrmann, J. F. Cara, L. Cuttler, L. L. Levitsky, and I. M. Rosenthal. "Ovarian hyperandrogenism as a

result of congenital adrenal virilizing disorders: evidence for perinatal masculinization of neuroendocrine function in women." *ACOG Current Journal Review* 3, no. 8 (1995): 27.

[106] Morishima, A. K. I. R. A., MELVIN M. Grumbach, EVAN R. Simpson, C. Fisher, and K. E. N. A. N. Qin. "Aromatase deficiency in male and female siblings caused by a novel mutation and the physiological role of estrogens." *The Journal of clinical endocrinology & metabolism* 80, no. 12 (1995): 3689-3698.

[107] Hogeveen, Kevin N., Patrice Cousin, Michel Pugeat, Didier Dewailly, Benoît Soudan, and Geoffrey L. Hammond. "Human sex hormone–binding globulin variants associated with hyperandrogenism and ovarian dysfunction." *The Journal of clinical investigation* 109, no. 7 (2002): 973-981.

[108] Sir-Petermann, Teresa, M. Maliqueo, B. Angel, H. E. Lara, F. Perez-Bravo, and S. E. Recabarren. "Maternal serum androgens in pregnant women with polycystic ovarian syndrome: possible implications in prenatal androgenization." *Human reproduction* 17, no. 10 (2002): 2573-2579.

[109] Hauth, John C., Rebecca G. Clifton, James M. Roberts, Leslie Myatt, Catherine Y. Spong, Kenneth J. Leveno, Michael W. Varner et al. "Maternal insulin resistance and preeclampsia." *American journal of obstetrics and gynecology* 204, no. 4 (2011): 327-e1.

[110] Mastrogiannis, Dimitrios S., Michail Spiliopoulos, Wadia Mulla, and Carol J. Homko. "Insulin resistance: the possible link between gestational diabetes mellitus and hypertensive disorders of pregnancy." *Current diabetes reports* 9, no. 4 (2009): 296.

[111] Hunter, A., S. Vimplis, A. Sharma, N. Eid, and W. Atiomo. "To determine whether first-degree male relatives of women with polycystic ovary syndrome are at higher risk of developing cardiovascular disease and type II diabetes mellitus." *Journal of Obstetrics and Gynaecology* 27, no. 6 (2007): 591-596.

[112] Gur, Esra Bahar, Muammer Karadeniz, and Guluzar Arzu Turan. "Fetal programming of polycystic ovary syndrome." *World journal of diabetes* 6, no. 7 (2015): 936.

[113] Melo, A. S., C. S. Vieira, M. A. Barbieri, A. C. J. S. Rosa-e-Silva, A. A. M. Silva, V. C. Cardoso, R. M. Reis, R. A. Ferriani, M. F. Silva-de-Sa, and H. Bettiol. "High prevalence of polycystic ovary syndrome in women born small for gestational age." *Human reproduction* 25, no. 8 (2010): 2124-2131.

[114] Ibáñez, Lourdes, Neus Potau, Inge Francois, and Francis de Zegher. "Precocious pubarche, hyperinsulinism, and ovarian hyperandrogenism in girls: relation to reduced fetal growth." *The Journal of Clinical Endocrinology & Metabolism* 83, no. 10 (1998): 3558-3562.

[115] Ibanez, L., J. E. Hall, N. Potau, A. Carrascosa, N. Prat, and A. E. Taylor. "Ovarian 17-hydroxyprogesterone hyperresponsiveness to gonadotropin-releasing hormone (GnRH) agonist challenge in women with polycystic ovary syndrome is not mediated by luteinizing hormone hypersecretion: evidence from GnRH agonist and human chorionic gonadotropin stimulation testing." *The Journal of Clinical Endocrinology & Metabolism* 81, no. 11 (1996): 4103-4107.

[116] Barker, David JP. "In utero programming of chronic disease." *Clinical science* 95, no. 2 (1998): 115-128.

[117] Ong, Ken K., and David B. Dunger. "Perinatal growth failure: the road to obesity, insulin resistance and cardiovascular disease in adults." *Best practice & research Clinical endocrinology & metabolism* 16, no. 2 (2002): 191-207.

[118] O'Brien, Jacob, Heyam Hayder, Yara Zayed, and Chun Peng. "Overview of microRNA biogenesis, mechanisms of actions, and circulation." *Frontiers in endocrinology* 9 (2018): 402.

[119] Condrat, Carmen Elena, Dana Claudia Thompson, Madalina Gabriela Barbu, Oana Larisa Bugnar, Andreea Boboc, Dragos Cretoiu, Nicolae Suciu, Sanda Maria Cretoiu, and Silviu Cristian Voinea. "miRNAs as biomarkers in disease: latest findings regarding their role in diagnosis and prognosis." *Cells* 9, no. 2 (2020): 276.

[120] López-Pastor, Andrea R., Jorge Infante-Menéndez, Óscar Escribano, and Almudena Gómez-Hernández. "miRNA Dysregulation in the

Development of Non-Alcoholic Fatty Liver Disease and the Related Disorders Type 2 Diabetes Mellitus and Cardiovascular Disease." *Frontiers in Medicine* 7 (2020).

[121] Butler, Alexandra E., Vimal Ramachandran, Thozhukat Sathypalan, Rhiannon David, Nigel J. Gooderham, Manasi Benurwar, Soha R. Dargham, Shahina Hayat, S. Hani Najafi-Shoushtari, and Stephen L. Atkin. "microRNA Expression in Women With and Without Polycystic Ovarian Syndrome Matched for Body Mass Index." *Frontiers in endocrinology* 11 (2020).

[122] Butler, Alexandra E., Vimal Ramachandran, Thomas Keith Cunningham, Rhiannon David, Nigel J. Gooderham, Manasi Benurwar, Soha R. Dargham et al. "Increased MicroRNA Levels in Women With Polycystic Ovarian Syndrome but Without Insulin Resistance: A Pilot Prospective Study." *Frontiers in endocrinology* 11 (2020): 754.

BIOGRAPHICAL SKETCH

Fouzia Rashid

Affiliation: Associate Professor, Clinical Biochemistry, University of Kashmir

Education:

- PhD Biochemistry, (Awarded 2005) Aligarh Muslim University, India.
- MSc Biochemistry, (2001) Aligarh Muslim University, India.
- BSc (Hon"s) Biochemistry, (1999) Aligarh Muslim University, India.

Research and Professional Experience: Metabolomics and Proteomics of Metabolic syndrome associated diseases including polycystic ovarian syndrome, diabetes.

Research Projects:

1. Quantitation and Comparative Evaluation of Insulin resistance, Pro-inflammatory and Pro- Coagulant Markers in Drug Naive versus Oral Contraceptive Pills (OCP'S) Treated PCOS Women. (DST, J & K)
2. Metabolic Evaluation of Oral Contraceptive (OCP's) Treated Polycystic Ovary Syndrome (PCOS) Women. (UGC, New Delhi)
3. Evaluation of genetic variants of ICAM-1, TNF-α, MCP-1, and PAI-1 gene in Kashmiri polycystic ovary syndrome (PCOS) women and Comparative expression analysis of these genes in drug naive versus oral contraceptive pills (OCP's) treated PCOS women. (DST- WOS-A)
4. Insulin Gene VNTR polymorphism in kashmiri women with polycystic ovary syndrome. (ICMR as Co-PI)
5. Expression analysis and polymorphism of CYP11, CYP17 and CYP19 genes and their relationship with hyper-androgenism and PCOS in Kashmiri women. (DHR as Co-PI)

Scientific Contributions:

The main focus of my research has been in metabolic profiling of metabolic syndrome associated disorders particularly Polycystic Ovarian Syndrome (PCOS). A number of projects mainly concerning PCOS have been executed with major contributions as under:

1. Long-term use of OCPs (Oral contraceptives) worsens Inflammatory and Coagulatory profile of women with several of their key markers like Adiponectin, Resistin, IL-1B, Visfatin,

ICAM, TNF-α, TF etc. showing significant variations. This study cautions against long-term use of OCPs.
2. OCP treatment also affects gene expression of several inflammatory genes like ICAM, TNF-α, MCP etc. when used over longer duration of time as we observed their increased m-RNA expression.
3. Altered PON1 enzyme activity and its polymorphism in PCOS put these women for future cardiovascular risk.
4. Deranged oxidative stress markers and enzymes in PCOS make these women susceptible to several stress borne diseases.
5. Elevated levels of Bisphenol A, an Endocrine disruptor, in PCOS women can lead to adverse pregnancy and neonatal outcomes.

Professional Appointments:

Position held	Institute Name	Duration Period
Assistant Professor	Clinical Biochemistry, University of Kashmir	2006 – 2018
Associate Professor	Clinical Biochemistry, University of Kashmir	2018 – till date

Honors: Young Scientist Award 2007, JKDST

Qualified All India Entrance test for CSIR/NET-JRF (June 2001)
Qualified All India Entrance test for ICMR-JRF (April 2001)
Qualified All India GATE (Graduate Aptitude test in Engineering) (Feb. 2001)

Publications from the Last 3 Years:

1. Humira Jeelani, Nahida Tabassum, Dil Afroze, Fouzia Rashid. Association of Paraoxonase1 enzyme and its genetic single nucleotide polymorphisms with cardio- metabolic and neurodegenerative diseases. https://doi.org/10.1016/j.genrep.2020.100775. *Gene Reports.* 2020.
2. Saika Manzoor, Mohd A. Ganie, Sabhiya Majid, Iram Shabir, Iram A. Kawa, Qudsia Fatima, Humira Jeelani, Syed Douhath Yousuf, Fouzia Rashid. Analysis of Intrinsic and Extrinsic

Coagulation Pathway Factors in OCP Treated PCOS Women. *Ind J Clin Biochem.* 2020. https://doi.org/10.1007/s12291-020-00901-w.

3. Jasiya Qadir, Sabhiya Majid, Mosin S. Khan, Fouzia Rashid, Mumtaz Din Wani, Inshah Din, Haamid Bashir. AT-rich Interaction Domain 1A Gene Variations: Genetic Associations and Susceptibility to Gastric Cancer Risk. *Pathology & Oncology Research.* 2020.

4. Sairish Ashraf, Shayaq Ul Abeer Rasool, Mudasar Nabi, Mohd Ashraf Ganie, Farhat Jabeen, Fouzia Rashid & Shajrul Amin. CYP17 gene polymorphic sequence variation is associated with hyperandrogenism in Kashmiri women with polycystic ovarian syndrome. *Gynecological Endocrinology.* 2020. DOI: 10.1080/09513590.2020.1770724.

5. Rasool SUA, Ashraf S, Nabi M, *Rashid F*, Fazili KM, Amin S. Elevated fasting insulin is associated with cardiovascular and metabolic risk in women with polycystic ovary syndrome. *Diabetes & metabolic syndrome: Clinical Research & Reviews.* 13(3), 20982105, 2019.

6. Rasool SUA, Ashraf S, Nabi M., *Rashid F*, Masoodi SR, Fazili KM. and Amin S. Insulin gene VNTR class III allele is a risk factor for insulin resistance in Kashmiri women with polycystic ovary syndrome. *Meta Gene.* 100597, 2019.

7. Rashid R, Geer MI, Verma SK, *Rashid F* and Ganaie A. Evaluation of prescription pattern and compliance in Kashmiri women with Polycystic Ovarian Syndrome. *Journal of Drug Delivery and Therapeutics.* 9(3), 379-383, 2019.

8. Saika Manzoor, Mohd Ashraf Ganie, Shajrul Amin, Zaffar A Shah, Imtiyaz A Bhat, S. Douhath Yousuf, Humira Jeelani, Iram A Kawa, Qudsia Fatima & *Fouzia Rashid*. Oral contraceptive use increases risk of inflammatory and coagulatory disorders in women with Polycystic Ovarian Syndrome: An observational study. *Scientific Reports.* 9, 10182, 2019.

9. Fatima Q, Amin S, Kawa IA, Jeelani J, Manzoor S, Rizvi SM, *Rashid F*. Evaluation of antioxidant defense markers in relation to hormonal and insulin parameters in women with polycystic ovary syndrome (PCOS): A case-control study. *Diabetes & Metabolic Syndrome: Clinical Research & Reviews.* 13, 1957-1961, 2019.
10. Ashaq I K, Masood A, Ganie MA, Fatima Q, Jeelani H, Manzoor S, Rizvi SM, Muzamil M, *Rashid F.* Bisphenol A (BPA) acts as an endocrine disruptor in women with Polycystic Ovary Syndrome: Hormonal and metabolic evaluation. *Obesity Medicine.* 14, 2451-8476, 2019.
11. Humira Jeelani, Mohd Ashraf Ganie, Akbar Masood, Shajrul Amin, Iram Ashaq Kawa, Qudsia Fatima, Saika Manzoor, Tabasum Parvez, Niyaz Ahmad Naikoo, Fouzia Rashid. Assessment of PON1 activity and circulating TF levels in relation to BMI, testosterone, HOMA-IR, HDL-C, LDL-C, CHO, SOD activity and TAC in women with PCOS: An observational study. *Diabetes & Metabolic Syndrome: Clinical Research & Reviews* 13 (2019) 2907-2915.
12. Jeelani H, Ganie. MA, Amin S, Fatima S, Ashaq I K, Manzoor S, Parvez T, Dar NA, *Rashid F.* Effect of Paraoxonase1 (PON1) gene polymorphisms on PON1 activity, HDL, LDL and MDA levels in women with polycystic ovary syndrome (PCOS): A case-control study. *Meta Gene,* 20,100552, 2019.
13. Nissar S, Sameer AS, Rasool R, Chowdri NA, *Rashid F.* Promoter methylation and Ile105Val polymorphism of GSTP1gene in modulation of colorectal cancer risk in ethnic kashmiri population. *Indian Journal of cancer,* 56; 248-53; 2019.
14. Douhath S, Ganie MA, Jeelani S, Mudassar S, Shah ZA, Zargar MA, Amin S, Wani IA & *Rashid. F.* Effect of six-month use of oral contraceptive pills on plasminogen activator inhibitor-1 & factor VIII among women with polycystic ovary syndrome: An observational pilot study. *Ind J Med Res.* 148 (7), 151-155, 2018.

15. Sairish A, Mudassir N, Shayeq R, *Rashid F,* Amin S. Hyperandrogenism in Polycystic ovarian syndrome and role of CYP gene variants: A review. *Egyptian Journal of Medical Human Genetics.* (Accepted Dec. 2018).

Books/Book Chapters:

1. Protein Misfolding Diseases: In *perspective of Gain and Loss of Function. 105-118. Proteostasis and Chaperone Surveillance,* Springer International, ISBN 97881-322- 2466-2. 2016.
2. Clinical perspective of post-translational modifications. 37-58, *Protein Modificomics*, Elsevier, ISBN: 978-0-12-811913-6. 2019.
3. Microbes in Reproductive tract spectrum: Inferences from microbial world, *Pathogenicity and drug resistance of human pathogens,* Springer International, ISBN 978981-329-449-3. 2019.

Chapter 3

POLYCYSTIC OVARY SYNDROME: A FRESH INSIGHT IN RELATION TO ITS INFLAMMATORY AND COAGULATORY PATHOPHYSIOLOGY

Saika Manzoor[1], Khalid Bashir Dar[1], Mohd Ashraf Ganie[2], Iram Ashaq Kawa[1] and Fouzia Rashid[1],*

[1]Department of Clinical Biochemistry/Biochemistry, University Of Kashmir, Srinagar, Jammu and Kashmir, India
[2]Department of Endocrinology and Metabolism, Sher-i-Kashmir Institute of Medical Sciences, Srinagar, Jammu and Kashmir, India

ABSTRACT

PCOS is a multi-factorial complex disorder affecting various organ systems of the body. It is a vicious cycle, when it gets triggered at any

---

* Corresponding Author's E-mail: rashid.fouzia@gmail.com.

unknown point; it results in full-blown metabolic syndrome. The diverse etiology of PCOS adversely affects various pathways like insulin resistance, lipid metabolism, steroidogenesis, inflammation, and coagulation cascade. Long-term risk factors associated with this disorder are T2DM, glucose intolerance, CVD, VTE, pulmonary embolism, infertility, pregnancy complications, cancer, etc. PCOS shoots beyond the scope of endocrine and reproductive abnormalities and is considered as a syndrome associated with metabolic dysfunctioning of the body. It can be considered, as an umbrella with a gallop of troubles underneath it. Therefore, its management requires collaborative efforts like lifestyle intervention i.e., eating habits, physical activities, use of medications, counseling, aesthetic approach and psychotherapies, etc. PCOS requires proper evaluation procedures to rule out its symptoms overlapping with other disease conditions. Various clinical symptoms that appear with the onset of disease are an indication of the underlying pathologies associated with PCOS. The main aim of this chapter is to provide an understanding and wider concept of pathogenesis and intricacy of various pathways pertaining to the heterogeneity of this syndrome that can help to comprehend the disease's progression in detail, especially in relation to the involvement of various inflammatory pathways and coagulatory disturbances which build up over time and can have serious implications for the overall health of the concerned individual. There is a crucial role of mechanisms like abnormal hypothalamus-pituitary-ovarian axis, hormonal imbalance, insulin resistance, hyperinsulinemia, deregulated production of inflammatory cytokines, and coagulatory factors in PCOS pathogenesis. Targeting these cascades for devising effective therapeutic management against such a far-reaching disorder could prove a beneficent strategy. Comprehensive knowledge added in this chapter will provide sufficient information pertaining to varied aspects of this disorder like various symptoms, different criteria, prevalence, reproductive, endocrine, cardiac, hematological, inflammatory, and coagulatory features, long-term outcomes, and the possible root causes of pathogenesis in this syndrome.

Keywords: coagulation cascade pathway, Factor V Leiden, hyperandrogenism, inflammation markers, metabolic syndrome, PCOS

INTRODUCTION

Human Polycystic Ovary Syndrome also called as Stein-Leventhal syndrome is not a recent disease in the medical era but it dates back to 1935 when the description of the polycystic ovaries was found associated with oligo/anovulation and hirsutism [1]. PCOS does not merely deal with the presence of cysts in the ovaries of the patients; it is a broader term in itself. PCOS includes metabolic as well as endocrine abnormalities of reproductive-age women. There is not a single common factor responsible for the PCOS etiology but it is a multifactorial disorder involving multiple organ systems of the body and thus includes a variety of clinical expression of varied etiological parameters. Different criteria are available regarding PCOS diagnoses like the National Institute of Health (NIH), Rotterdam, and Androgen Excess-PCOS Society (AES-PCOS). The NIH conference was first held in the year 1990 regarding the diagnostic criteria of PCOS, sponsored by the United States. It is also known as "classical PCOS" that includes two criteria i.e., hyperandrogenism (clinical as well as biochemical) and menstrual irregularities with the exclusion of different disorders that may resemble PCOS in their manifestations like Cushing's syndrome, late-onset congenital adrenal hyperplasia, androgen-secreting tumors etc [2]. However, in the year 2003, the European Society for Human Reproduction & Embryology (ESHRE) and the American Society for Reproductive Medicine (ASRM) included one more feature in its diagnostic criteria i.e., the ultra-sonographic description of polycystic ovarian morphology in these women. Hence, the present-day Rotterdam criteria is the result of revised ESHRE/ ASRM, which includes the presence of two out of three features i.e., hyperandrogenism (clinical as well as biochemical), menstrual irregularities, and typical ultra-sonographic appearance of the ovaries [3]. Moreover, in the year 2006, the Androgen Excess Society (AES) now called as Androgen Excess and PCOS Society (AE-PCOS) provided the third definition of PCOS diagnosis, which emphasizes the presence of hyperandrogenism as an essential feature for its diagnostic criteria. Hence, according to AES-PCOS diagnostic criteria - the presence of hyperandrogenism is considered as an ultimate feature of PCOS while any of the other two features i.e., menstrual irregularity or ultra-sonographic description of polycystic ovaries can be considered for its diagnosis [4]. There is a prevalence of 4-10% according to NIH criteria, however, its prevalence is greater according to Rotterdam criteria i.e., about 3-26% as is described in Figure 1 [5-8].

The duration of the normal menstrual cycle in most women ranges between 21 to 35 days while as in the case of menstrual irregularity, cycles are shorter than 21 days and longer than 35 days. It includes abnormal blood flow as well as dysmenorrhea [9, 10]. The prevalence of menstrual irregularity in PCOS women has been reported to be 14.6% to 22.8% [11].

Various signs and symptoms associated with this disorder include the absence of a menstrual cycle, infertility, poor body image like facial hair growth, obesity, alopecia and acne, which affects the overall quality of life in these women. All these contributing factors lead to psychopathology and impaired emotional well-being that results in the higher prevalence of psychiatric disorders like anxiety, depression, social fears, and suicidal tendency in these women [12]. Stress is considered as the main factor for these psychiatric disorders and anxiety is the most common disorder found in PCOS women [13].

There is the huge economic burden of PCOS worldwide i.e., about 4 billion dollars are spent in the United States for screening and treatment of this disease while as Australian Health System spends 800 million dollars annually in this regard [14]. However, statistical data are scarce regarding the prevalence of PCOS in India due to the heterogeneity of PCOS criteria followed pertaining to its diagnosis. Thorough management is required to reduce the overall economic cost and burden caused by this disorder.

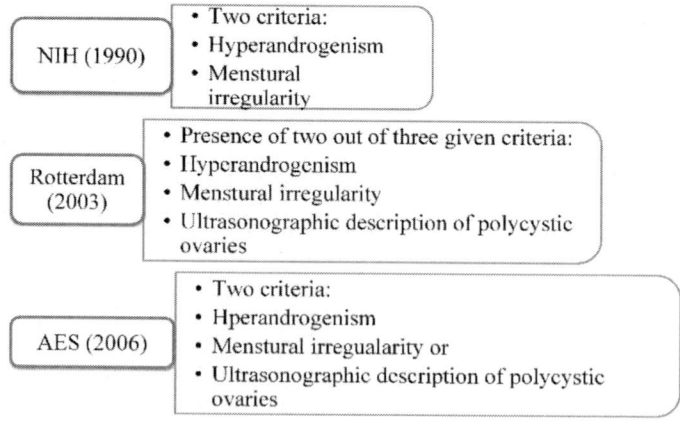

Figure 1. Guidelines for the diagnosis of PCOS.

METABOLIC SPECTRUMS AND PCOS

The prevalence of the metabolic syndrome is 33% in PCOS women. According to National Cholesterol Education Program (NCEP), metabolic syndrome can be defined as involvement of abnormalities in parameters like fasting glucose, blood pressure, waist circumference, and lipid metabolism specific to triglycerides and HDL cholesterol [15]. However, an earlier definition of WHO included insulin resistance as essential criteria for consideration of metabolic syndrome [16]. Moreover, long-term outcomes of metabolic syndrome such as Type 2 diabetes mellitus (T2DM), CVD, cancers, hypertension, insulin resistance, dyslipidemia, and obesity are considered as associated risk factors in PCOS conditions as well. Since, the conditions associated with the metabolic syndrome are prevalent in PCOS, therefore, these pathological conditions i.e., metabolic syndrome and PCOS are overlapping with each other.

HYPERANDROGENISM AND PCOS

Hyperandrogenism is defined as androgen excess, which is clinically manifested in form of acne, male-pattern alopecia, and hirsutism while hyperandrogenemia refers to increased androgen levels in blood circulation. Hyperandrogenism is considered as the key feature of PCOS and the prevalence of its clinical manifestation is as: 15-25% acne, 65-75% hirsutism and 5-50% androgenic alopecia [11].

There is a common steroidogenic pathway for androgen formation in ovaries as well as in adrenal glands. Normally, ovaries secrete 60% of androgens in response to LH. The LH production causes stimulation of theca cells of the ovaries, which results in the synthesis of ovarian androgens like DHEA and androstenedione [17, 18] while 40% of androgens are secreted in response to ACTH by adrenal glands. However, in the case of PCOS women, there is an increased pulsatile LH level that causes the increased synthesis of ovarian androgen production that circulates freely in the blood.

The increased androgen levels do not provide a negative feedback mechanism on LH production in these females.

Under normal physiological conditions, stimulation of the adrenal cortex by ACTH causes the production of adrenal androgens. However, in PCOS women there is an increased ACTH production due to dysfunction of the Hypothalamic-Pituitary-Adrenal axis (HPA) that increases the stimulation of the adrenal cortex, ultimately causing elevation of adrenal androgen production in these women.

Hence, the overall hypothalamic-pituitary-ovarian axis abnormality in PCOS women results in the increased secretion of LH and ACTH from their respective glands that causes increased androgen production and their bioavailability which affects the overall steroidogenesis pathway in these women as is described in Figure 2.

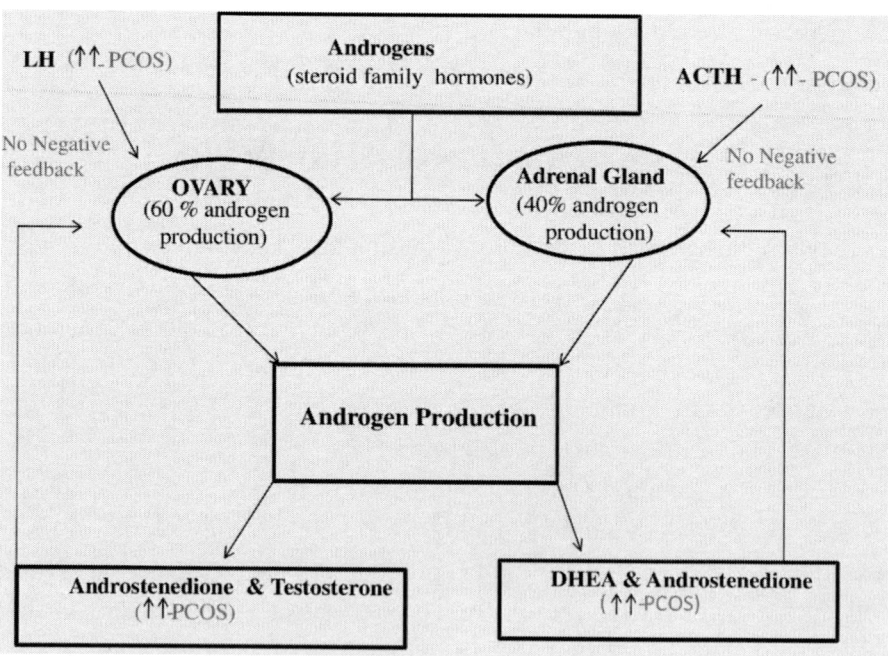

Figure 2. Steroidogenesis pathway in PCOS women.

INSULIN RESISTANCE AND PCOS

Insulin is a hormone that is known to play an important role in the normal regulation of the body's metabolism. It causes glycogenesis i.e., conversion of glucose into glycogen hence, lowering the blood glucose levels and causes lipogenesis as well. However, IR is an impaired metabolic condition where in spite of having normal insulin concentrations in the body, it does not produce normal insulin response in various target tissues and there is no absolute reduction of blood glucose levels [19]. As a result, pancreatic beta cells produce compensatory hyperinsulin to maintain glucose levels within normal ranges. With the progression of time, pancreatic beta cells tend to deteriorate and thus prevent lowering of glucose that result in glucose intolerance and eventually may lead to T2DM, if left untreated.

It has been observed that various steps are involved in the normal insulin signaling pathway like glucose uptake, inhibition of lipolysis, increased expression, and translocation of GLUT-4 but these are reported to be decreased in women with PCOS [20-23]. Insulin signaling operates by two important pathways namely AKT/PI-3K and MAPK pathway. When the insulin binds to its receptor, it causes phosphorylation of insulin receptor substrates (IRS1 & IRS 2). An effector molecule known as PI-3K recognizes the phosphorylated IRS1 and hence causes phosphorylation of AKT. The AKT-a key player in insulin metabolism is known to cause phosphorylation of AS160, which in turn causes activation of GLUT-4 that result in glucose uptake by insulin stimulation. However, in PCOS women, it has been reported that protein phosphatases are activated by free fatty acids. These phosphatases cause dephosphorylation of the AKT that cannot further activate AS160 and results in GLUT-4 inactivation and therefore no glucose uptake. The decreased glucose uptake and GLUT-4 expression have been linked with the defects in AKT/PI-3K pathway in PCOS women.

Hyperinsulinemia plays a central role in the pathogenesis of PCOS and is considered the main candidate for hyperandrogenism. Insulin resistance over sensitizes the theca cells of the ovaries to LH response and also causes decreased synthesis of SHBG by the liver which otherwise binds to the free testosterone [24, 25]. The steroidogenic pathway for the synthesis of androgens under normal physiological as well as in PCOS conditions is diagrammatically summarized in Figure 3.

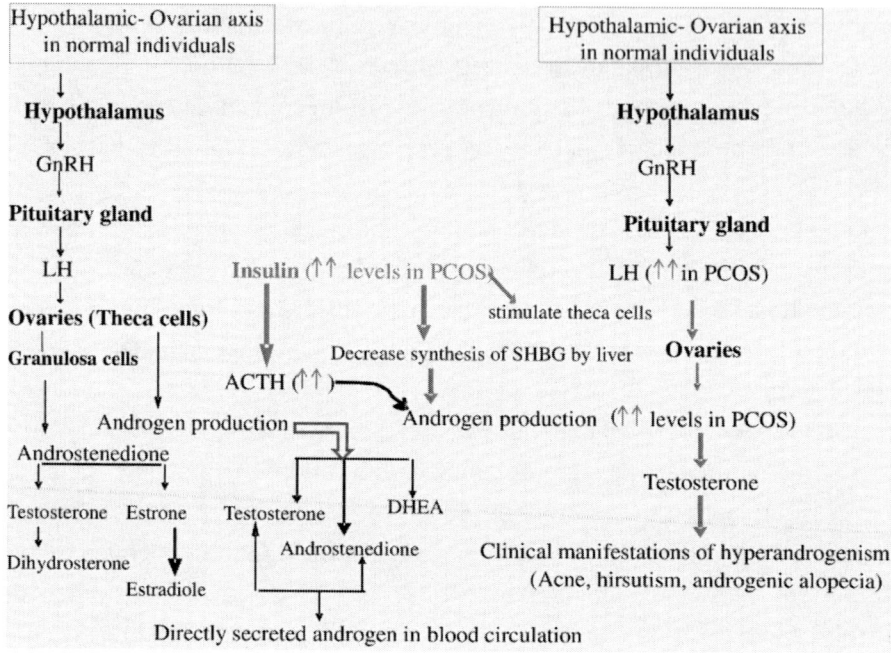

Figure 3. Steroidogenic pathway for the synthesis of androgens under normal physiological as well as in PCOS conditions.

Clinical manifestation of IR in PCOS women is the presence of acanthosis nigricans i.e., dark velvety patches that can be seen on the groin, armpits, neck, joints of the fingers, and toes. Euglycemic clamp technique is considered the most consistent method for measurement of IR but is costly and time-consuming. Therefore, other simpler methods like insulin tolerance test can be employed for this purpose but are not considered much reliable as that of euglycemic clamp technique [26]. Moreover, IR in women with PCOS is known to suppress lipolysis which causes recruitment of excess fat from the adipose tissues thus alters the normal lipid profile that causes dyslipidemia in these women. Dyslipidemia has been found associated with atherogenesis and impairment in the coagulation cascade pathway. Hence,

IR plays a key role in the causation of metabolic derangements in PCOS women and therefore predisposes them to various risk factors like glucose intolerance, T2DM, CVD, and clotting disorders [19].

DYSLIPIDEMIA AND PCOS

Women with PCOS posseses various metabolic aberrations like IR, hyperandrogenism, hormonal imbalance, obesity and increased waist-hip ratio that tends to alter the normal lipid metabolic pathway and plays a contributing role in the causation of dyslipidemia in these women. Different patterns of dyslipidemia have been observed in these women and most commonly reported is low HDL cholesterol and high triglyceride levels [27, 28]. A highly susceptible risk factor with dyslipidemia is an increased waist-hip ratio as the central fat of the body is highly resistant to the insulin that promotes lipolysis to provide more availability of free fatty acids [29, 30].

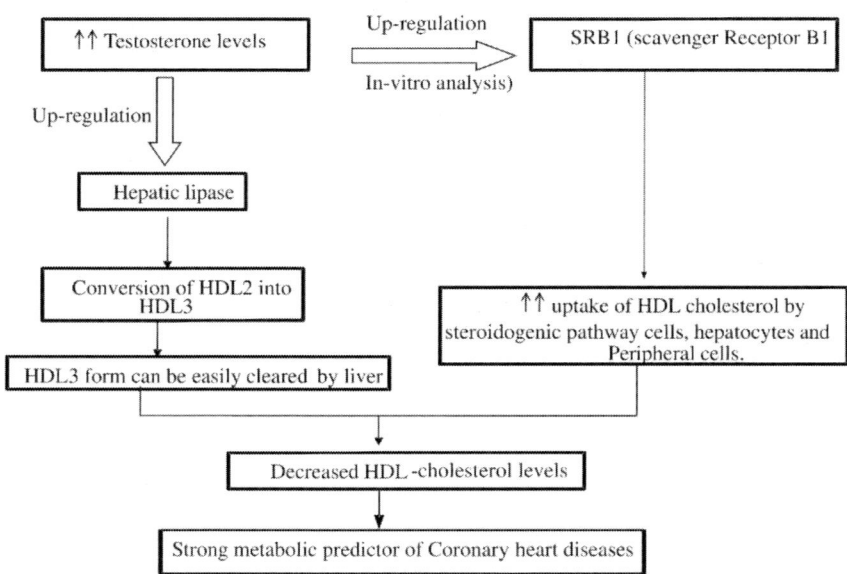

Figure 4. Diagrammatical representation of hyperandrogenism effect on lipid metabolism.

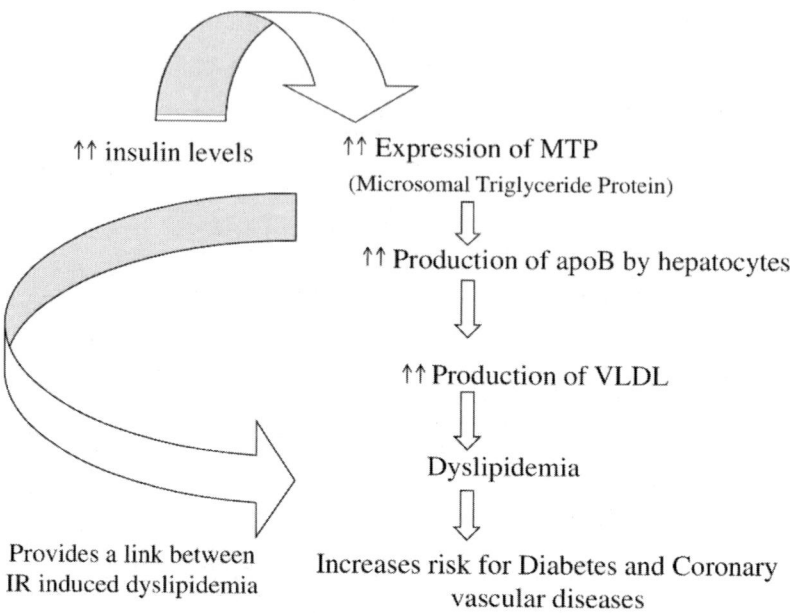

Figure 5. Diagrammatical presentation of hyperinsulinemia effect on lipid metabolism.

Moreover, hyperandrogenism is also known to affect the lipid metabolic pathway as it lowers the good cholesterol levels i.e., HDL cholesterol in these women. In-vitro studies have provided insight regarding the various possibilities that could explain how hyperandrogenism is responsible for dyslipidemia. It has been reported that testosterone causes up-regulation of two genes namely scavenger receptor B1 (SR-B1) and hepatic lipase (HL). Upregulation of SRB1 gene has been shown to cause uptake of HDL cholesterol by cells of the steroidogenic pathway, hepatocytes and peripheral cells while as HL catalyzes the conversion of HDL_2 into HDL_3 which can be easily cleared by liver in this form as described in Figure 4 [31-33].

Another important concept that could explain the linkage between hyperinsulinemia and dyslipidemia is the aberration of the apo-B (ligand of LDL-receptor) mechanism. Under normal physiological conditions, insulin is known to down-regulate the expression of microsomal triglyceride protein (MTP) while as in the case of hyperinsulinemia MTP expression is enhanced that increases the production of apoB by hepatocytes (as is described in Figure 5) which in turn causes increased production of VLDL subsequently

[34, 35]. Although there is not any specific mechanism known yet that could explain dyslipidemia in this syndrome, however, all the above-mentioned factors somehow contribute to the abnormal lipid profile in these women.

INFLAMMATION AND PCOS

Inflammation is an immune response to various diseases and is linked with metabolic deregulations like insulin resistance, hyperandrogenism, obesity, and dyslipidemia [36]. Deranged metabolic profile is common in women with PCOS and is thus, considered as chronic low-grade inflammatory disorder [37]. It is not clear yet whether inflammation is a cause or consequence of PCOS [38].

Hyperglycemia is considered as one of the key factors responsible for causing inflammation in PCOS women. Mononuclear cells (MNCs) in the blood circulation normally utilize the glucose molecules to produce NADPH, which gets oxidized to ROS due to activation of membrane-bound NADPH oxidase. ROS-induced oxidative stress ultimately leads to the activation of a transcription factor called NF-KB, which gets translocated to the nucleus to promote the expression of various pro-inflammatory mediators like IL-6 and TNF-α [39, 40]. TNF-α is also known to be a mediator of insulin resistance. Hence, the hyperglycemic condition prevailing in PCOS women causes an increase in inflammation as well as oxidative stress in this syndrome. Oxidative stress induced by ROS causes endothelial dysfunctioning, which may show its manifestation in the form of CVD and hypertension [41]. Thus, insulin resistance and PCOS result in a suitable milieu for inflammation and its associated co-morbidities.

Hyperandrogenism, one of the hallmarks of PCOS pathogenesis is known to promote inflammation in PCOS women. Hyperandrogenism enhances the production of pro-inflammatory cytokine TNF-α by increasing the sensitization of MNCs to glucose [42]. Moreover, in vitro analysis has shown that pro-inflammatory stimuli like TNF-α cause elevated production of androgen levels by increasing the stimulation of androgen-producing theca cells of the ovaries [43]. Inflammation, in turn, may promote hyperandrogenism in PCOS as well. Therefore, these studies show that there is a definite link between hyperandrogenism and inflammation.

Earlier it was proposed that elevated inflammatory markers were found associated with obesity conditions only, as adipocyte hypertrophy modifies macrophages into pro-inflammatory cells, which increases the pro-inflammatory cytokine production [38, 44]. Essentially, hypertrophic conditions result in the compression of the stromal vessels which causes activation of transcription factor nuclear factor kappa B (NF-KB) that mediates pro-inflammation markers like hs-CRP, interleukins (IL-β, IL-6, IL-10, IL-18), cell adhesion molecules (VCAM, ICAM), transforming growth factor β (TGF-β), monocyte chemotactic protein -1 (mcp-1) and TNF α which further recruits macrophages and sustain inflammation for longer period time [45]. However, elevated levels of pro-inflammatory cytokines are being observed in lean as well as in obese PCOS individuals. Therefore, it is suggestive of an independent association of inflammation with PCOS [46, 47]. Since, a strong correlation between pro-inflammatory markers like ILs, CRP has been reported with CVD and atherosclerosis. Thus PCOS women are at greater risk of developing these diseases [44]. Various pro-inflammatory cytokines that are found to be elevated in PCOS women; some of them are discussed as under:

Adiponectin

Adiponectin is an anti-inflammatory adipocytokine produced predominantly by adipocytes. Its expression is found down regulated during obese conditions [48]. This cytokine is also found to possess anti-insulin and anti-atherogenic actions that have deeper implications in PCOS conditions [49, 50]. There are two receptors for adiponectin protein namely AdipoR1 and AdipoR2, which are expressed in skeletal muscles and hepatocytes respectively whose ligand binding results in the activation of AMPK and PPAR-α. AMPK activation helps in the oxidation of fatty acids, increases NO production in endothelial cells while PPAR-α reduces liver steatosis and enhances insulin sensitivity. Adiponectin increases phosphorylation and activation of AMPK, elevation in NO production, increase in glucose uptake, reduction in gluconeogenesis, prevention of both TNF-α induced monocytes adhesion to endothelial cells and TNF-α induced NF-KB activation [51]. Hence, the reduction in adiponectin level affects the normal physiological functioning of the system associated with its expression and thus increases the risk of various diseases like hyperinsulinemia, endothelial dysfunctioning, coagulation abnormalities, atherosclerosis, and inflammation [52].

Interleukin-1beta (IL-1β)

It is a member of the IL family which consists of a family of 11 cytokines and is an effective pro-inflammatory mediator produced by activated macrophages that plays an important role in defense responses to injury and infection [53]. Pro-IL-1β is activated by pro-caspase1, which in turn gets activated by the inflammasome and forms an activated IL1-β whose binding to interleukin 1 receptor (IL-1R) causes intracellular signaling [54]. IL-1β plays a role in female reproduction processes like ovulation and oocyte maturation, inflammatory-linked mechanisms such as production and activation of proteolytic enzymes, prostaglandin production, nitric oxide production, and steroidogenesis [55, 56]. IL-1β plays an important role in other normal physiological conditions as well like homeostasis, renal, hepatic functioning, hematopoiesis, regulation of blood pressure, sleep, ACTH release, and increased sodium excretion [57, 58]. It is also known to play a role in lipid metabolism by regulating insulin levels and lipase activity under physiological conditions [59]. Elevated levels of IL-1β are linked not only to various autoimmune and auto-inflammatory diseases but also to metabolic deregulations. The subsequent abnormal secretion of this cytokine is associated with type II diabetic and impaired beta-cell function [60, 61]. Rather than being directly cytotoxic, IL-1β drives tissue inflammation that impacts both beta-cell functional mass and insulin sensitivity in type 2 diabetes [62]. Hence, the over-production of IL-1 β is found associated with various disease conditions like inflammation, vascular diseases, atherosclerosis, chronic heart failure, and T2DM, which are considered as, associated risk factors for PCOS [63].

Visfatin

Visfatin is an important pro-inflammatory cytokine secreted from adipocytes, bone marrow, fetal membranes, liver, muscles, trophoblasts, lymphocytes, and hepatocytes. It causes the elevation of various other cytokines like TNF-α, IL-6, and IL-1β. It also increases cell adhesion molecules such as ICAM, VCAM that recruit leucocytes which interferes with the inflammatory pathways [64]. Glucose and insulin levels are considered as the main regulators of visfatin, hence, the levels of visfatin get increased in hyperglycemic and low HDL-cholesterol conditions [65]. Visfatin is known to possess an insulin-mimetic effect that causes uptake of glucose by adipocytes and muscles as it causes phosphorylation of insulin receptor, insulin receptor substrate 1 and 2 (IRS1 &IRS2) subsequently by AMP kinase activity [66]. It is known to cause increased expression of GLUT4 and its translocation as well hence increases insulin sensitivity by binding to insulin receptors [67]. Visfatin levels are raised in various metabolic disorders like obesity, insulin resistance, and T2DM, which are well-known risk factors for PCOS [68].

Resistin

An important adipocytokine secreted by adipocytes, macrophages, spleen, bone marrow, and mononuclear cells (PBMCs) is remarkably implicated in insulin resistance. However, the mechanism is still not clear. It plays an important role in IR, obesity, autoimmune disorders, inflammation, thrombosis, and endothelial dysfunctions that are all related to PCOS pathophysiology [69, 70]. A Study performed by Steppan and co-workers showed that resistin administration impairs glucose uptake by adipocytes, which leads to IR. Similarly, administration of anti-resistin antibodies in obese and IR mice resulted in increased sensitivity of insulin [71]. These results indicate that resistin plays a definite role in decreasing insulin sensitivity promoting IR, thus predisposing to T2DM.

Resistin levels also show an elevation in response to stimuli like TNF-α, IL-6, and lipopolysaccharides (LPS) that trigger production of various inflammatory cytokines. It is believed to bind membrane-bound Toll Like Receptor 4 (TLR4), which in turn triggers the intracellular signaling pathways leading to inflammation. It causes translocation of NF-Kβ into the nucleus and activates transcription of various pro-inflammatory cytokines. All these contributing factors indicate a potential role of resistin in promoting inflammation. It also promotes ROS generation, which inhibits eNOS and NOS production [72]. The later is implicated in endothelial dysfunctioning, thrombosis, and atherosclerosis, which are among the risk factors of PCOS. Furthermore, resistin is also implicated in the increase of 17-α hydroxylase that plays an important role in promoting hyperandrogenism, a key factor for PCOS pathogenesis [73]. Overall, it seems that resistin has a multidimensional role in various pathophysiologies linked directly or indirectly with PCOS.

Peroxisome Proliferator-Activated Receptor Gamma (PPARγ)

There is an interesting correlation between PPARγ and PCOS as PPARγ is known to play a diverse role in various processes like insulin signaling, glucose uptake, immune cell activation, inflammation, and adipogenesis and is presented diagrammatically as under (as is described in Figure 6).

PPARγ is primarily expressed in ovaries, immune cells, and adipose tissues and gets activated naturally by the various ligands called polyunsaturated fatty acids (PUFAs) like $\omega 3$- and $\omega 6$.

Several mechanisms are involved in the regulation of insulin sensitization and glucose uptake through PPARγ which includes-

- Increased GLUT-4 expression
- Increased phosphatidyl-3-kinase activity

- Elevated phosphorylation of insulin receptor and insulin receptor substrates
- Reduction of PAI-1, TNF-α and free fatty acid (FFA).

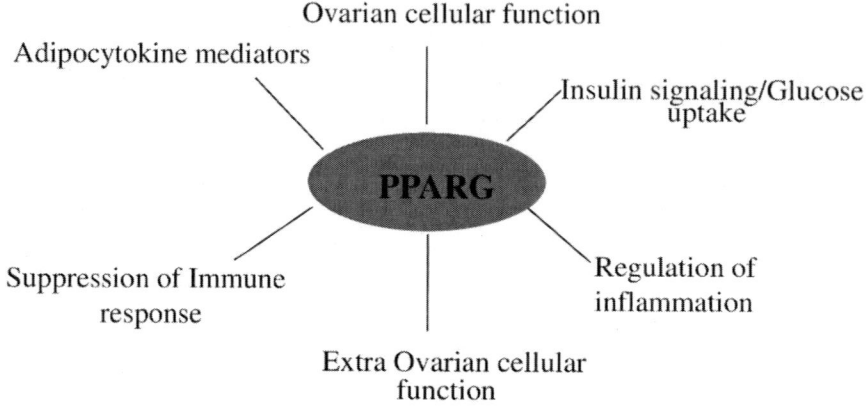

Figure 6. Diverse roles of PPARγ in various processes.

Ovarian macrophages are regulated by steroidogenesis as well as by gonadotropins required for the physiological functioning of various events like folliculogenesis, ovulation and reproductive functions. An increased population of immune cells under the influence of LH surge in theca cells of the ovary in pre-ovulation phase causes increased production of inflammatory cells, which are required to breakdown the epithelial lining of the ovary and maintain higher levels of PPARγ in ovarian cells. This scenario causes elevated levels of PPARγ in non-ovarian cells as well where it acts as an anti-inflammatory in action. Since there are receptors for various adipocytokines like leptin and adiponectin in the ovary of females and PPARγ is known to cause regulation of these adipocytokines. PPARγ is known to regulate the steroidogenesis pathway by decreasing the levels of leptin and acts as an anti-inflammatory agent by increasing the levels of adiponectin [74]. Therefore, there is a definite link between PPARγ and the female reproductive system. Thus, PPARγ can be considered as a good target to reverse the aberration associated with PCOS condition by increasing the activity of PPARγ using artificial ligand activation e.g., thiazolidinedione (TZD) treatment.

In our earlier reports, we have analyzed various anti and pro-inflammatory cytokines like Adiponectin, Interleukin 1β, Visfatin, and Resistin in drug-naive Polycystic Ovary Syndrome (PCOS) women versus oral contraceptive pills (OCPs) treated women. Decreased levels of anti-inflammatory marker (adiponectin) i.e., hypo-adiponectinaemia were observed in OCP-treated PCOS subjects compared to drug-naive PCOS subjects. However, elevated levels of pro-inflammatory cytokines like interleukin1β, visfatin and resistin were observed in OCP-treated PCOS subjects compared to drug-naive PCOS subjects. This data regarding anti and pro-inflammatory cytokines is suggestive of negative effects of oral contraceptives in PCOS women and agrees with the various studies as reported elsewhere [75].

COAGULATION CASCADE AND PCOS

The Coagulation cascade pathway is a complex process that involves the formation of blood clots in response to injury under the action of blood clotting factors to prevent excessive blood loss from the body. This pathway involves both the formation as well as dissolution of clots that requires the balanced amount of coagulant and anti-coagulant components to maintain a proper hemostatic system. Imbalance in these components may result in coagulation disorders that cause impairment in the body's ability to control the clotting mechanism. Generally, clot formation results in thrombosis (i.e., obstruction to blood flow), however, disseminated intravascular coagulation (DIC) characterized by widespread/uncontrolled hypercoagulable state involves increased intravascular clot formation that often ruptures thereby causing hemorrhages i.e., increase in bleeding [76]. Thrombosis is a pathological condition that involves the presence of clots in the heart as well as in other blood vessels. Hypercoagulability plays a crucial role in thrombosis, which may result in venous thromboembolism (VTE). VTE is a broader term that includes other severe conditions like deep vein thrombosis (DVT) and pulmonary embolism (PE). DVT is a condition with an abnormal clot that occludes in deep veins, usually in the legs while PE involves the breakdown of the clot that may travel to the lungs and prevents the blood supply. It can be symptomatic like tenderness, leg pain, and shortness of breath or it could be asymptomatic as well. VTE is considered the third most common cause of CVD in the general population [77-79].

Various coagulation factors mentioned below are known to play an important role in the maintenance of blood homeostasis and regulate the associated pathological conditions. One of the key factors in the coagulation pathway is factor V, produced by the liver. It is also known as proaccelerin or liable factor and is present as an inactive pro-coagulant molecule in the blood circulation while 20% of total protein is present within α granule [80, 81]. It gets activated as factor Va in response to specific stimuli like the injury to blood vessels. The activated Factor V (FVa) forms a complex with the factor Xa, which causes the conversion of inactive protein component, called pro-thrombin into active component called thrombin. Thrombin causes clot formation by causing the conversion of fibrinogen into fibrin [82]. Another remarkable property of FV is its ability to bind with the natural anti-coagulant i.e., Activated Protein C (APC) to prevent excessive clot formation in the system. APC is a natural anti-coagulant of both Factor V and FVIIIa which shuts off the clot formation plot in the body. Inactivation of FVa by APC occurs by the cleavage of FV at three different amino acid positions 306, 506 & 679 Arginine. Hence, FV possesses dual functionality i.e., acts as a coagulant as well as an anti-coagulant. Consequently, FVa plays a crucial role in the maintenance of clot formation tendency to prevent hypercoagulability and prevents excess blood loss from the system as well.

Tissue factor also called as factor III is mainly expressed in blood cells, few examples being monocytes, macrophages, granulocytes, and platelets [83]. Tissue factor initiates extrinsic blood coagulation which proceeds as Ca^{2+} dependent extracellular signaling and results in the activation of following factors-FVII, FX, and prothrombin (FII): FVIIa, FXa and FIIa respectively. Activated factor II (FIIa) cleaves off fibrinogen into fibrin monomers that cross-links to produce insoluble blood clots. The intrinsic pathway merges with tissue factor initiates the coagulation pathway at FX activation (FXa) step [84-86]. Circulating tissue factor levels are found to be elevated in women with PCOS independent of obesity that leads to a thrombotic state in these women. Moreover, a higher concentration of tissue factor has been found within atheromatous plaque as compared to surrounding tissues [87]. Rupturing of plaque exposes tissue factor to the circulating blood, thus, it triggers thrombosis and occludes blood vessels [88, 89].

Prothrombin time (PT) and activated partial thromboplastin time (APTT) are important clinical parameters for assessing extrinsic and intrinsic factors/pathways of the coagulation system [90]. Prothrombin time (PT) gives an indication of the concentration of prothrombin in the blood. Thus, PT measures the time taken for fibrin formation or coagulation time through the extrinsic pathway. The normal value of PT is about 12 seconds. Activated Partial Thromboplastin Time (APTT) is a measurement of the intrinsic coagulation pathway. It measures the time taken for fibrin formation through the intrinsic pathway, usual values being 25-36 seconds. Shortened PT and APTT values reflect a hypercoagulable state, which may result from the accumulation of circulating activated coagulation factors present in the plasma, which is potentially associated with increased thrombotic risk and adverse cardiovascular events [91-94].

Tissue plasminogen activator (tPA) is an important key factor of the fibrinolytic system, which converts inactive plasminogen into active plasmin. Plasmin acts on fibrin fibers of the clot causing its depolarization and thus results in clot dissolution. It also helps in the inactivation of the clotting cascade pathway by causing hydrolysis of various pro-coagulants like FV, VIII, and XI [95]. Elevated levels of tPA have been observed in women with PCOS that indicates the underlying pathophysiological condition at play which tends to increase its levels in these women. Although, tPA is responsible for excess clot removal that otherwise may occlude blood circulation pathway; at the same time it points towards coagulopathy, being one of the upshots of the disease process. Furthermore, a strong inverse correlation has been established between tPA and insulin sensitivity while, no correlation has been observed with testosterone [96, 97]. Figure 7 shows the molecular cascade associated with clot formation and degradation.

D-dimer is not normally present in the plasma of human blood but its presence is the confirmation of activated coagulation cascade pathway. Thus, the elevated D-dimer levels are an indication of thrombosis that results due to secondary fibrinolysis [98]. D-dimer is the end product of fibrin degradation and its elevated levels have been observed in PCOS individuals [99, 100]. Elevated levels of both the fibrinolytic components like tPA and D-dimer is a savior pathway that prevents the excess clot formation in the system, but their elevated levels at the same time reveal a hypercoagulability state in these women. PCOS is considered, as a hypercoagulable state although the exact mechanism responsible for PCOS induced hypercoagulability is not clear; it is likely due to heterogeneous responses like insulin resistance, hyperandrogenism and hormonal imbalance.

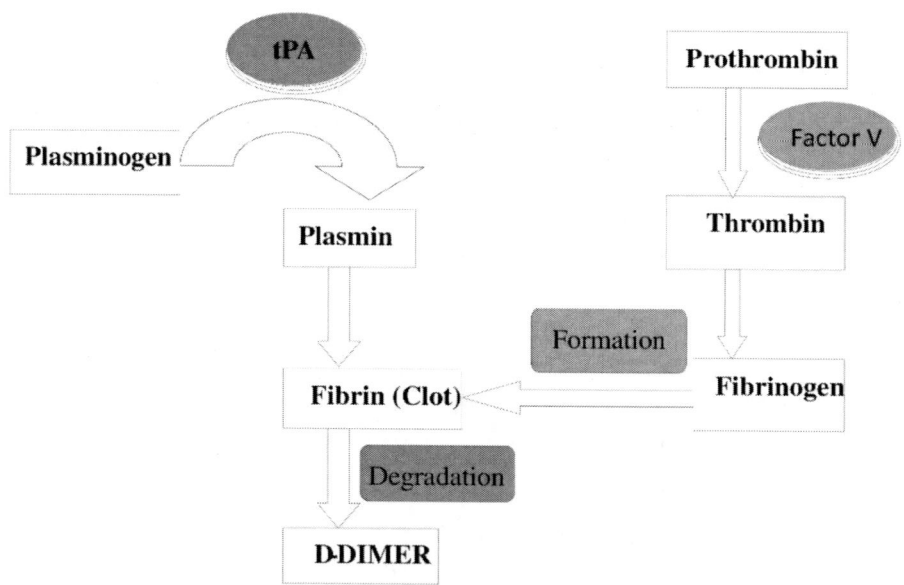

Figure 7. Diagrammatical presentation of clot formation and degradation.

Hyperinsulinemia that plays a key role in PCOS etiology is known to decrease the synthesis of SHBG that may result in enhanced secretion of fibrinolysis inhibitor factor PAI-1. Hence the insulin resistance results in increased thrombus formation in these women and hyperglycemia is reported to enhance pro-coagulation which results in hypercoagulability

[101]. Thus, the activation of the coagulation cascade pathway increases the susceptibility of various other disease processes like CVD in this syndrome [102, 103]. It has been reported there is a two-fold risk of VTE in PCOS women and this risk is further elevated in OCP users [104].

There are only a few studies available that have reported a link between hyperandrogenism and coagulation cascade in PCOS conditions [105]. It has been found that insulin-sensitizing drugs cause decreased levels of coagulation factor PAI-1 that consequently down-regulates the levels of testosterone with the drug treatment suggesting a possible link between androgen levels and coagulation factors in PCOS [106].

The previous work in our lab about the effect of oral contraceptive mode of treatment in PCOS women has shown adverse outcomes on the coagulatory profile of these women. The various pro-coagulatory markers assessed in our study included Tissue factor, PT, APTT, Factor XI, Factor V, TAT III complex, tPA and D-dimer. All the mentioned coagulation parameters analyzed in our study reflected the hypercoagulable state in these women [75].

FACTOR V LEIDEN AND PCOS

Hypercoagulable state can arise due to genetic as well as acquired conditions i.e., either a person has inherited a tendency to form clots or it is acquired due to trauma or other medical conditions. Women with PCOS are reported to have three times more familial history of venous thrombosis than the general population [107]. Apart from the concentration of various pro and anti-coagulants, genetic inheritance could be one of the major aspects of thrombophilia (multiple clot formation tendencies) [108].

One of the important factors that contribute to the inherited thrombophilia is Factor V Leiden. Factor V Leiden is a name proposed for specific gene mutation and is named after the Dutch investigator, from the city of Leiden, who first reported it. Factor V Leiden is a single nucleotide mutation at 1691 nucleotide of FV gene, which causes the substitution of glutamine for arginine at 506 (R506Q) APC cleavage site. The FV Leiden mutation causes the inactivation of Factor VIIIa, which further exacerbates the pro-thrombotic status in the system. Hypercoagulability caused by FVL mutation arises due to resistance of Factor V to natural anticoagulant APC that is unable to inactivate factor V normally which keeps the clot formation pathway active for a longer period time that ultimately results in the thrombophilia [109].

Factor V Leiden diagnosis can be done in two different ways i.e., APC resistance test and DNA analysis method [110]. There is a wide range of variation regarding the clinical aspect of this mutation, which ranges from the individuals with no thrombosis to frequent development of VTE at the age of fewer than 30 years. However, the clinical manifestation of this mutation is VTE [111, 112]. It has been estimated that approximately 30% of individuals with VTE developed recurrent thrombosis [113]. Moreover, the risk of recurrent VTE in the case of FV Leiden is found higher in heterozygous individuals as compared to homozygous individuals [114]. There are 3-8 folds increased risk of VTE in heterozygote's while 10-80 folds increased thrombotic risk has been reported in homozygotes [115, 116]. It has been reported that about 20%-60% of excess clot formation i.e., thrombophilia found in Caucasians is reported due to factor V point mutation called FVL mutations (Factor V Leiden), which involves the substitution of arginine by glutamine at 506 [117]. Apart from the thrombotic risk associated with FV Leiden mutation, it has been reported that there is an increased risk of pregnancy loss with this mutation [110]. Placental thrombosis is attributed to the complications like infertility and miscarriages associated with Factor V Leiden [118]. Moreover, a link between thrombophilia and miscarriages is an indication of the predisposition of PCOS women to increased risk of thrombosis due to FV. It is postulated that women with PCOS may experience the conditions associated with thrombophilia due to endocrinopathies associated with PCOS [119]. Furthermore, large meta-analysis studies have reported a link between FV Leiden and Coronary vascular diseases (CVD). It has been reported that FVL increases the risk for myocardial infarctions, strokes, and arterial thrombotic events [120].

All the above-mentioned complications associated with Factor V Leiden mutation like hypercoagulability, miscarriages, infertility, DVT, VTE and CVD (as is described in Figure 8) are associated co-morbidities found in women with PCOS as well. Therefore, the screening of these women for Factor V Leiden might be helpful to assess the risk factors associated with the coagulation cascade pathway in these women.

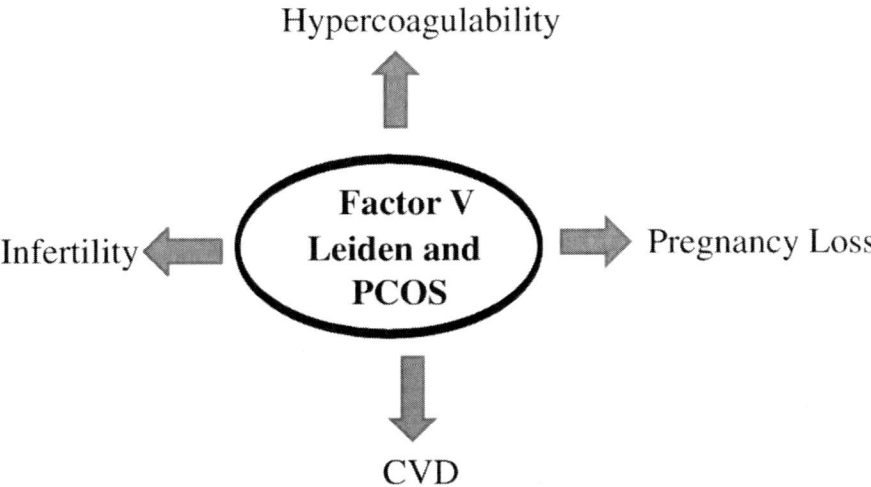

Figure 8. Complications associated with Factor V Leiden mutation in PCOS women.

PSYCHOLOGICAL DISORDERS AND PCOS

The vulnerability of PCOS women to psychiatric disorders is not well understood. However, stress is considered as one of the major contributing factors that induce psychological disorders in this syndrome. Abnormal hypothalamic-pituitary-adrenal dysfunctioning disrupts the normal neuroendocrine functionality and shows an adverse impact on health resulting in the stress-related co-morbidities in this syndrome. Another aspect is androgen metabolic deregulation, which is considered responsible for the psychiatric disorders in this syndrome. Associated co-morbidities with PCOS like infertility, acne and hirsutism are also found associated with decreased mental well-being in these women [12]. There is a wide range of psychiatric disorders in PCOS women which includes depression, anxiety, obsessive-compulsive disorder, bipolar, eating disorders, somatization, social phobia and panic disorders [121].

Depression can be defined as the lowering of mood that remains deeper and persistent. According to NIH, depression affects about 5% of the population per year and 13% of the population during their whole life. The majority of population with depressive disorders possesses suicidal tendencies and one-third of them attempt suicide. The frequency of depression is most common between the age of 20 and 40 years and is more prevalent in females compared to males. A literature survey made by Accortt and co-workers from the year 1965 to 2008 has shown the prevalence of depression is twice in females compared to males [122]. Moreover, it has been reported that there is a seven-fold increased risk of suicidal tendencies in PCOS women [123]. Among various depressive disorders, fatigue and sleeping disorders are considered the most common ones with the prevalence of 96% and 88% respectively.

Anxiety being the psychological disorder that runs parallel to depression in this syndrome and is reported to have a prevalence of 34% in women with PCOS in a study conducted by Benson and co-workers [124]. The various complications associated with this syndrome like acne, infertility, obesity and elevated testosterone levels are found to be PCOS-associated outcomes responsible for depression and anxiety [125]. Hence, PCOS women are at an increased risk of both depressive as well as anxiety disorders. There is uncertainty regarding the relationship between bipolar disorders (i.e., the alternate occurrence of mania and depression) and PCOS because there is only 1% occurrence of this disorder in the general population. However, women are more prone to it [126]. Moreover, there is an ambiguity regarding the association between PCOS and eating disorders. A study by Michelmore et al. reported no association between PCOS and eating disorders [127]. While in another study, 36.3% of the women with eating disorders belonged to the PCOS group only [128]. Overall, there is low quality of life in these women due to low self-esteem, poor body image and hirsutism followed by other psychological distress [129]. Thus, early screening and proper treatment strategies need to be followed that helps to reduce the risk of various psychiatric disorders associated with this syndrome [130].

CONCLUSION

PCOS affects multiple functioning of the body including reproductive, endocrine, cardiac, hematological, and psychological processes. It can be considered as an umbrella with a gallop of troubles underneath it and therefore, its management requires collaborative efforts like lifestyle intervention i.e., eating habits, physical activities, use of medications, counseling, aesthetic approach and psychotherapies, etc. PCOS is much complex in the inference of both pathogenesis and outcome thus each patient needs to be treated carefully. Every patient differs from others in terms of symptoms and severity of the disorder. Therefore, an adequate individual treatment approach should be provided to the patients keeping all the complications into consideration rather than generalizing the same treatment plan for all PCOS women. It requires proper evaluation procedures to rule out as its symptoms overlap with other disease conditions. Various clinical symptoms that appear with the onset of disease are an indication of the underlying processes associated with PCOS. If the symptoms of PCOS are not addressed at the earliest, there can be the adverse long-term outcomes of the disease and can further exacerbate into full-blown metabolic syndrome.

In this chapter, we tried to emphasize various pathways involved in PCOS development, to provide a better understanding of the pathogenesis and progression of this disorder. Subsequently, this review highlights the role of crucial mechanisms like abnormal hypothalamus-pituitary-ovarian axis, hormonal imbalance, IR, hyperinsulinemia, deregulated production of inflammatory cytokines (Adiponectin, Interleukin 1β, Visfatin, Resistin and PPARγ), and coagulatory factors (Tissue factor, PT, APTT, FXI, Factor V, D-dimer, tPA, and Thrombin-antithrombin III (TAT-III complex) in PCOS pathogenesis. Thus, it pinpoints the need to target these cascades for devising effective therapeutic management against such a far-reaching disorder. Moreover, extensive literature survey and research need to be done in this regard to provide better insight for proper understanding and treatment of the diseases.

REFERENCES

[1] Stein, Irving F. "Amenorrhea associated with bilateral polycystic ovaries." *American Journal of Obstetrics and Gynecology* 29 (1935): 181-191.

[2] Zawadzski, J. K. "Diagnostic criteria for polycystic ovary syndrome: towards a rational approach." *Polycystic Ovary Syndrome* (1992): 39-50.

[3] Welt, C. K., J. A. Gudmundsson, G. Arason, J. Adams, H. Palsdottir, G. Gudlaugsdottir, G. Ingadottir, and W. F. Crowley. "Characterizing discrete subsets of polycystic ovary syndrome as defined by the Rotterdam criteria: the impact of weight on phenotype and metabolic features." *The Journal of Clinical Endocrinology and Metabolism* 91, no. 12 (2006): 4842-4848.

[4] Azziz, Ricardo, Enrico Carmina, Didier Dewailly, EvanthiaDiamanti-Kandarakis, Hector F. Escobar-Morreale, Walter Futterweit, Onno E. Janssen et al. "Criteria for defining polycystic ovary syndrome as a predominantly hyperandrogenic syndrome: an androgen excess society guideline." *The Journal of Clinical Endocrinology and Metabolism* 91, no. 11 (2006): 4237-4245.

[5] Azziz, Ricardo, Keslie S. Woods, Rosario Reyna, Timothy J. Key, Eric S. Knochenhauer, and Bulent O. Yildiz. "The prevalence and features of the polycystic ovary syndrome in an unselected population." *The Journal of Clinical Endocrinology & Metabolism* 89, no. 6 (2004): 2745-2749.

[6] Hashemipour, Mahin, MassoudAmini, RaminIranpour, GholamHossein Sadri, NargesJavaheri, SassanHaghighi, Silva Hovsepian, Abbas Ali Javadi, Mahdi Nematbakhsh, and GoshtasbSattari. "Prevalence of congenital hypothyroidism in

Isfahan, Iran: results of a survey on 20,000 neonates." *Hormone Research in Paediatrics* 62, no. 2 (2004): 79-83.

[7] Driscoll, Deborah A. "Polycystic ovary syndrome in adolescence." In *Seminars in Reproductive Medicine*, vol. 21, no. 03, pp. 301-308. Copyright© 2003 by Thieme Medical Publishers, Inc., 333 Seventh Avenue, New York, NY 10001, USA. Tel.:+ 1 (212) 584-4662, 2003.

[8] Eshre, The Rotterdam, and ASRM-Sponsored PCOS Consensus Workshop Group. "Revised 2003 consensus on diagnostic criteria and long-term health risks related to polycystic ovary syndrome." *Fertility and Sterility* 81, no. 1 (2004): 19-25.

[9] American College of Obstetricians and Gynecologists. "ACOG practice bulletin no. 127: Management of preterm labor." *Obstetrics and Gynecology* 119, no. 6 (2012): 1308-1317.

[10] Whitaker, Lucy, and Hilary OD Critchley. "Abnormal uterine bleeding." *Best Practice & Research Clinical Obstetrics and Gynaecology* 34 (2016): 54-65.

[11] Azziz, Ricardo, Enrico Carmina, Didier Dewailly, EvanthiaDiamanti-Kandarakis, Héctor F. Escobar-Morreale, Walter Futterweit, Onno E. Janssen et al. "The Androgen Excess and PCOS Society criteria for the polycystic ovary syndrome: the complete task force report." *Fertility and Sterility* 91, no. 2 (2009): 456-488.

[12] Sayyah-Melli, Manizheh, MahastiAlizadeh, NosratollahPourafkary, ElahehOuladsahebmadarek, MehriJafari-Shobeiri, JalehAbbassi, Maryam alsadatKazemi-Shishvan, and Kamran Sedaghat. "Psychosocial factors associated with polycystic ovary syndrome: A case control study." *Journal of Caring Sciences* 4, no. 3 (2015): 225.

[13] Sonino, Nicoletta, Cecilia Navarrini, Chiara Ruini, FedraOttolini, AgostinoPaoletta, Francesco Fallo, Marco Boscaro, and Giovanni A. Fava. "Persistent psychological distress in patients treated for endocrine disease." *Psychotherapy and Psychosomatics* 73, no. 2 (2004): 78-83.

[14] Azziz, Ricardo, Catherine Marin, LalimaHoq, EnkheBadamgarav, and Paul Song. "Health care-related economic burden of the polycystic ovary syndrome during the reproductive life span." *The*

Journal of Clinical Endocrinology and Metabolism 90, no. 8 (2005): 4650-4658.

[15] Expert Panel on Detection, Evaluation. "Executive summary of the third report of the National Cholesterol Education Program (NCEP) expert panel on detection, evaluation, and treatment of high blood cholesterol in adults (Adult Treatment Panel III)." *JAMA* 285, no. 19 (2001): 2486.

[16] Alberti, Kurt George Matthew Mayer, and Paul Z. Zimmet. "Definition, diagnosis and classification of diabetes mellitus and its complications. Part 1: diagnosis and classification of diabetes mellitus. Provisional report of a WHO consultation." *Diabetic medicine* 15, no. 7 (1998): 539-553.

[17] Wood, Jennifer R., and Jerome F. Strauss. "Multiple signal transduction pathways regulate ovarian steroidogenesis." *Reviews in Endocrine and Metabolic Disorders* 3, no. 1 (2002): 33-46.

[18] Jamnongjit, Michelle, and Stephen R. Hammes. "Ovarian steroids: the good, the bad, and the signals that raise them." *Cell Cycle* 5, no. 11 (2006): 1178-1183.

[19] ManzoorSaika, Mohd Ashraf Ganie, S. DouhathYousuf, Shajrul Amin, Habib R, Fouzia Rashid. Metabolic derangements and possible CVD risk in PCOS women owing to use of OCP's as a treatment mode – pros and cons. *Diabetes, Obesity and Metabolism* 2017; 5:1109.

[20] Dunaif, Andrea, Xinqi Wu, Anna Lee, and EvanthiaDiamanti-Kandarakis. "Defects in insulin receptor signaling in vivo in the polycystic ovary syndrome (PCOS)." *American Journal of Physiology-Endocrinology and Metabolism* 281, no. 2 (2001): E392-E399.

[21] Diamanti-Kandarakis, Evanthia, and Athanasios G. Papavassiliou. "Molecular mechanisms of insulin resistance in polycystic ovary syndrome." *Trends in Molecular Medicine* 12, no. 7 (2006): 324-332.

[22] Dunaif, Andrea, Jinru Xia, Carol-Beth Book, Esther Schenker, and Zhichun Tang. "Excessive insulin receptor serine phosphorylation in cultured fibroblasts and in skeletal muscle. A potential mechanism for

insulin resistance in the polycystic ovary syndrome." *The Journal of Clinical Investigation* 96, no. 2 (1995): 801-810.
[23] Li, Ming, Jack F. Youngren, Andrea Dunaif, Ira D. Goldfine, Betty A. Maddux, Bei B. Zhang, and Joseph L. Evans. "Decreased insulin receptor (IR) autophosphorylation in fibroblasts from patients with PCOS: effects of serine kinase inhibitors and IR activators." *The Journal of Clinical Endocrinology & Metabolism* 87, no. 9 (2002): 4088-4093.
[24] Baptiste, Catherine G., Marie-Claude Battista, AndréanneTrottier, and Jean-Patrice Baillargeon. "Insulin and hyperandrogenism in women with polycystic ovary syndrome." *The Journal of Steroid Biochemistry and Molecular Biology* 122, no. 1-3 (2010): 42-52.
[25] Rosenfield, Robert L., and David A. Ehrmann. "The pathogenesis of polycystic ovary syndrome (PCOS): the hypothesis of PCOS as functional ovarian hyperandrogenism revisited." *Endocrine Reviews* 37, no. 5 (2016): 467-520.
[26] Bernier, Danielle. *Polycystic Ovary Syndrome: Pathogenesis, health consequences, and treatment of PCOS in relation to insulin resistance.* (2012).
[27] Meirow, Dror, ItamarRaz, OferYossepowitch, Amnon Brzezinski, Ariel Rosler, G. Schenker, and Elliot Berry. "Dyslipidaemia in poly cystic ovarian syndrome: different groups, different aetiologies?." *Human Reproduction* 11, no. 9 (1996): 1848-1853.
[28] Yilmaz, Murat, Aydan Biʻriʻ, NeslihanBukan, AyhanKarakoç, BanuSancak, FüsunTörüner, and HaticePaşaoğlu. "Levels of lipoprotein and homocysteine in non-obese and obese patients with polycystic ovary syndrome." *Gynecological Endocrinology* 20, no. 5 (2005): 258-263.
[29] Yildirim, Basak, NuranSabir, and Babur Kaleli. "Relation of intra-abdominal fat distribution to metabolic disorders in nonobese patients with polycystic ovary syndrome." *Fertility and Sterility* 79, no. 6 (2003): 1358-1364.

[30] Mittelman, Steven D., Gregg W. Van Citters, Erlinda L. Kirkman, and Richard N. Bergman. "Extreme insulin resistance of the central adipose depot in vivo." *Diabetes* 51, no. 3 (2002): 755-761.

[31] Kozarsky, Karen F., Mary H. Donahee, Jane M. Glick, Monty Krieger, and Daniel J. Rader. "Gene transfer and hepatic overexpression of the HDL receptor SR-BI reduces atherosclerosis in the cholesterol-fed LDL receptor–deficient mouse." *Arteriosclerosis, Thrombosis, and Vascular Biology* 20, no. 3 (2000): 721-727.

[32] Langer, Claus, Barbara Gansz, Christian Goepfert, Thomas Engel, Yoshinari Uehara, Gerlinde von Dehn, Hans Jansen, GerdAssmann, and Arnold von Eckardstein. "Testosterone up-regulates scavenger receptor BI and stimulates cholesterol efflux from macrophages." *Biochemical and biophysical Research Communications* 296, no. 5 (2002): 1051-1057.

[33] Herbst, Karen L., John K. Amory, John D. Brunzell, Howard A. Chansky, and William J. Bremner. "Testosterone administration to men increases hepatic lipase activity and decreases HDL and LDL size in 3 wk." *American Journal of Physiology-Endocrinology and Metabolism* 284, no. 6 (2003): E1112-E1118.

[34] Wetterau, John R., M. C. Lin, and Haris Jamil. "Microsomal triglyceride transfer protein." *BiochimicaetBiophysicaActa* 1345, no. 2 (1997): 136-150.

[35] Taghibiglou, Changiz, André Carpentier, Stephen C. Van Iderstine, Biao Chen, Debbie Rudy, Andrea Aiton, Gary F. Lewis, and KhosrowAdeli. "Mechanisms of hepatic very low density lipoprotein overproduction in insulin resistance: evidence for enhanced lipoprotein assembly, reduced intracellular ApoB degradation, and increased microsomal triglyceride transfer protein in a fructose-fed hamster model." *Journal of Biological Chemistry* 275, no. 12 (2000): 8416-8425.

[36] Hotamisligil, Gökhan S. "Inflammation and metabolic disorders." *Nature* 444, no. 7121 (2006): 860-867.

[37] Shorakae, Soulmaz, Helena Teede, Barbora de Courten, Gavin Lambert, Jacqueline Boyle, and Lisa J. Moran. "The emerging role of

chronic low-grade inflammation in the pathophysiology of polycystic ovary syndrome." In *Seminars in Reproductive Medicine*, vol. 33, no. 04, pp. 257-269. Thieme Medical Publishers, 2015.

[38] Carmina, E. (2013). Obesity, adipokines and metabolic syndrome in polycystic ovary syndrome. *Polycystic Ovary Syndrome*, *40*, 40-50.

[39] Piotrowski, P. C., I. J. Rzepczynska, J. Kwintkiewicz, and A. J. Duleba. "Oxidative stress induces expression of CYP11A, CYP17, star and 3 beta HSD in rat theca-interstitial cells." In *Journal of the Society for Gynecologic Investigation*, vol. 12, no. 2, pp. 319A-319A. 360 Park Ave South, New York, NY 10010-1710 USA: Elsevier Science INC, 2005.

[40] Gambineri, A., C. Pelusi, V. Vicennati, U. Pagotto, and R. Pasquali. "Obesity and the polycystic ovary syndrome." *International Journal of Obesity* 26, no. 7 (2002): 883-896.

[41] Hulsmans, Maarten, and Paul Holvoet. "The vicious circle between oxidative stress and inflammation in atherosclerosis." *Journal of Cellular and Molecular Medicine* 14, no. 1-2 (2010): 70-78.

[42] González, Frank. "Inflammation in polycystic ovary syndrome: underpinning of insulin resistance and ovarian dysfunction." *Steroids* 77, no. 4 (2012): 300-305.

[43] Spaczynski, Robert Z., Aydin Arici, and Antoni J. Duleba. "Tumor necrosis factor-α stimulates proliferation of rat ovarian theca-interstitial cells." *Biology of Reproduction* 61, no. 4 (1999): 993-998.

[44] Wisse, Brent E. "The inflammatory syndrome: the role of adipose tissue cytokines in metabolic disorders linked to obesity." *Journal of the American Society of Nephrology* 15, no. 11 (2004): 2792-2800.

[45] Spritzer, Poli Mara, Sheila B. Lecke, FabíolaSatler, and Debora M. Morsch. "Adipose tissue dysfunction, adipokines, and low-grade chronic inflammation in polycystic ovary syndrome." *Reproduction* 149, no. 5 (2015): R219-R227.

[46] Ebejer, Krystle, and Jean Calleja-Agius. "The role of cytokines in polycystic ovarian syndrome." *Gynecological Endocrinology* 29, no. 6 (2013): 536-540.

[47] Samy, Nervana, MahaHashim, Magda Sayed, and Mohamed Said. "Clinical significance of inflammatory markers in polycystic ovary syndrome: their relationship to insulin resistance and body mass index." *Disease Markers* 26, no. 4 (2009): 163-170.

[48] Carmina, E., M. C. Chu, R. A. Longo, G. B. Rini, and R. A. Lobo. "Phenotypic variation in hyperandrogenic women influences the findings of abnormal metabolic and cardiovascular risk parameters." *The Journal of Clinical Endocrinology & Metabolism* 90, no. 5 (2005): 2545-2549.

[49] Weyer, Christian, P. Antonio Tataranni, Clifton Bogardus, and Richard E. Pratley. "Insulin resistance and insulin secretory dysfunction are independent predictors of worsening of glucose tolerance during each stage of type 2 diabetes development." *Diabetes care* 24, no. 1 (2001): 89-94.

[50] Kadowaki, Takashi, and Toshimasa Yamauchi. "Adiponectin and adiponectin receptors." *Endocrine reviews* 26, no. 3 (2005): 439-451.

[51] Whitehead, J. P., A. A. Richards, I. J. Hickman, G. A. Macdonald, and J. B. Prins. "Adiponectin–a key adipokine in the metabolic syndrome." *Diabetes, Obesity and Metabolism* 8, no. 3 (2006): 264-280.

[52] Dıez, Juan J., and Pedro Iglesias. "The role of the novel adipocyte-derived hormone adiponectin in human disease." *European Journal of endocrinology* 148, no. 3 (2003): 293-300.

[53] Dinarello, Charles A. *Biologic basis for interleukin-1 in disease.* (1996): 2095-2147.

[54] Ren, Ke, and Richard Torres. "Role of interleukin-1β during pain and inflammation." *Brain research reviews* 60, no. 1 (2009): 57-64.

[55] Gérard, Nadine, Maud Caillaud, Alain Martoriati, GhylèneGoudet, and Anne-Christine Lalmanach. "The interleukin-1 system and female reproduction." *Journal of Endocrinology* 180, no. 2 (2004): 203-212.

[56] Caillaud, Maud, Guy Duchamp, and Nadine Gérard. "In vivo effect of interleukin-1beta and interleukin-1RA on oocyte cytoplasmic

maturation, ovulation, and early embryonic development in the mare." *Reproductive biology and endocrinology* 3, no. 1 (2005): 1-9.

[57] Crown, John, Ann Jakubowski, and Janice Gabrilove. "Interleukin-1: biological effects in human hematopoiesis." *Leukemia and lymphoma* 9, no. 6 (1993): 433-440.

[58] Malarkey, William B., and Bharathi J. Zvara. "Interleukin-1β and other cytokines stimulate adrenocorticotropin release from cultured pituitary cells of patients with Cushing's disease." *The Journal of Clinical Endocrinology and Metabolism* 69, no. 1 (1989): 196-199.

[59] Matsuki, Taizo, Reiko Horai, KatsukoSudo, and YoichiroIwakura. "IL-1 plays an important role in lipid metabolism by regulating insulin levels under physiological conditions." *The Journal of experimental medicine* 198, no. 6 (2003): 877-888.

[60] Mandrup-Poulsen, T., K. Bendtzen, J_ Nerup, C. A. Dinarello, M. Svenson, and J. H. Nielsen. "Affinity-purified human interleukin I is cytotoxic to isolated islets of Langerhans." *Diabetologia* 29, no. 1 (1986): 63-67.

[61] Eizirik, Décio L. "Interleukin-1 induced impairment in pancreatic islet oxidative metabolism of glucose is potentiated by tumor necrosis factor." *European Journal of Endocrinology* 119, no. 3 (1988): 321-325.

[62] Ehses, J.A., Lacraz, G., Giroix, M.H., Schmidlin, F., Coulaud, J., Kassis, N., Irminger, J.C., Kergoat, M., Portha, B., Homo-Delarche, F. and Donath, M.Y., 2009. IL-1 antagonism reduces hyperglycemia and tissue inflammation in the type 2 diabetic GK rat. *Proceedings of the National Academy of Sciences*, *106*(33), pp.13998-14003.

[63] Maedler, Kathrin, GitanjaliDharmadhikari, Desiree M. Schumann, and Joachim Størling. "Interleukin-1 beta targeted therapy for type 2 diabetes." *Expert opinion on biological therapy* 9, no. 9 (2009): 1177-1188.

[64] Kim, Su-Ryun, Yun-HeeBae, Soo-Kyung Bae, Kyu-Sil Choi, Kwon-Ha Yoon, Tae Hyeon Koo, Hye-Ock Jang et al. "Visfatin enhances ICAM-1 and VCAM-1 expression through ROS-dependent NF-κB

activation in endothelial cells." *BiochimicaetBiophysicaActa (BBA)-Molecular Cell Research* 1783, no. 5 (2008): 886-895.

[65] Hug, Christopher, and Harvey F. Lodish. "Visfatin: a new adipokine." *Science* 307, no. 5708 (2005): 366-367.

[66] Xie, H., S. Y. Tang, X. H. Luo, J. Huang, R. R. Cui, L. Q. Yuan, H. D. Zhou, X. P. Wu, and E. Y. Liao. "Insulin-like effects of visfatin on human osteoblasts." *Calcified Tissue International* 80, no. 3 (2007): 201-210.

[67] Haider, D. G., G. Schaller, S. Kapiotis, C. Maier, A. Luger, and M. Wolzt. "The release of the adipocytokinevisfatin is regulated by glucose and insulin." *Diabetologia* 49, no. 8 (2006): 1909-1914.

[68] Chang, Yu-Hung, Dao-Ming Chang, Kun-Cheng Lin, Shyi-Jang Shin, and Yau-Jiunn Lee. "Visfatin in overweight/obesity, type 2 diabetes mellitus, insulin resistance, metabolic syndrome and cardiovascular diseases: a meta-analysis and systemic review." *Diabetes/Metabolism Research and Reviews* 27, no. 6 (2011): 515-527.

[69] Konrad, Astrid, Michael Lehrke, VeronikaSchachinger, Frank Seibold, Renee Stark, Thomas Ochsenkühn, Klaus G. Parhofer, BurkhardGöke, and Uli C. Broedl. "Resistin is an inflammatory marker of inflammatory bowel disease in humans." *European Journal of Gastroenterology & Hepatology* 19, no. 12 (2007): 1070-1074.

[70] Gnacińska, M., S. Małgorzewicz, M. Stojek, W. Łysiak-Szydłowska, and K. Sworczak. "Role of adipokines in complications related to obesity. A review." *Advances in Medical Sciences (De Gruyter Open)* 54, no. 2 (2009).

[71] Steppan, Claire M., Elizabeth J. Brown, Christopher M. Wright, SavithaBhat, Ronadip R. Banerjee, Charlotte Y. Dai, Gregory H. Enders et al. "A family of tissue-specific resistin-like molecules." *Proceedings of the National Academy of Sciences* 98, no. 2 (2001): 502-506.

[72] Jamaluddin, Md S., Sarah M. Weakley, Qizhi Yao, and Changyi Chen. "Resistin: functional roles and therapeutic considerations for cardiovascular disease." *British Journal of Pharmacology* 165, no. 3 (2012): 622-632.

[73] Munir, Iqbal, Hui-Wen Yen, Talia Baruth, RafalTarkowski, Ricardo Azziz, Denis A. Magoffin, and Artur J. Jakimiuk. "Resistin stimulation of 17α-hydroxylase activity in ovarian theca cells in vitro: relevance to polycystic ovary syndrome." *The Journal of Clinical Endocrinology and Metabolism* 90, no. 8 (2005): 4852-4857.

[74] Minge, Cadence E., Rebecca L. Robker, and Robert J. Norman. "PPAR gamma: coordinating metabolic and immune contributions to female fertility." *PPAR Research* 2008 (2008).

[75] ManzoorSaika, Mohd Ashraf Ganie, Shajrul Amin, Zaffar A. Shah, Imtiyaz A. Bhat, S. DouhathYousuf, HumiraJeelani, Iram A. Kawa, Qudsia Fatima, and Fouzia Rashid. "Oral contraceptive use increases risk of inflammatory and coagulatory disorders in women with Polycystic Ovarian Syndrome: an observational study." *Scientific Reports* 9, no. 1 (2019): 1-8.

[76] Papageorgiou, C., Jourdi, G., Adjambri, E., Walborn, A., Patel, P., Fareed, J., Elalamy, I., Hoppensteadt, D and Gerotziafas, G.T. "Disseminated intravascular coagulation: an update on pathogenesis, diagnosis, and therapeutic strategies." *Clinical and Applied Thrombosis/Hemostasis* 24(9_suppl): 2018: 8S-28S.

[77] Giuntini, Carlo, Giorgio Di Ricco, Carlo Marini, Elio Melillo, and Antonio Palla. "Epidemiology." *Chest* 107, no. 1 (1995): 3S-9S.

[78] Næss, Inger Anne, S. C. Christiansen, P. Romundstad, S. C. Cannegieter, Frits R. Rosendaal, and Jens Hammerstrøm. "Incidence and mortality of venous thrombosis: a population‐based study." *Journal of thrombosis and Haemostasis* 5, no. 4 (2007): 692-699.

[79] Raskob, Gary E., Roy Silverstein, Dale W. Bratzler, John A. Heit, and Richard H. White. "Surveillance for deep vein thrombosis and pulmonary embolism: recommendations from a national workshop." *American Journal of Preventive Medicine* 38, no. 4 (2010): S502-S509.

[80] Rosing, Jan, and Guido Tans. "Coagulation factor V: an old star shines again." *Thrombosis and Haemostasis* 78, no. 07 (1997): 427-433.

[81] Alberio, L., O. Safa, Kenneth John Clemetson, C. T. Esmon, and G. L. Dale. "Surface expression and functional characterization of α-granule factor V in human platelets: effects of ionophore A23187, thrombin, collagen, and convulxin." *Blood, the Journal of the American Society of Hematology* 95, no. 5 (2000): 1694-1702.

[82] Kane, William H., Jozef S. Mruk, and Philip W. Majerus. "Activation of coagulation factor V by a platelet protease." *The Journal of clinical investigation* 70, no. 5 (1982): 1092-1100.

[83] Key, Nigel S., and Nigel Mackman. "Tissue factor and its measurement in whole blood, plasma, and microparticles." In *Seminars in Thrombosis and Hemostasis*, vol. 36, no. 08, pp. 865-875. © Thieme Medical Publishers, 2010.

[84] Chu, Arthur J. "Tissue factor mediates inflammation." *Archives of Biochemistry and Biophysics* 440, no. 2 (2005): 123-132.

[85] Furie, Bruce, and Barbara C. Furie. "Mechanisms of thrombus formation." *New England Journal of Medicine* 359, no. 9 (2008): 938-949.

[86] Butenas, Saulius, Thomas Orfeo, and Kenneth G. Mann. "Tissue factor activity and function in blood coagulation." *Thrombosis Research* 122 (2008): S42-S46.

[87] Marmur, Jonathan D., Singanallore V. Thiruvikraman, Billie S. Fyfe, ArabindaGuha, Samin K. Sharma, John A. Ambrose, John T. Fallon, Yale Nemerson, and Mark B. Taubman. "Identification of active tissue factor in human coronary atheroma." *Circulation* 94, no. 6 (1996): 1226-1232.

[88] Manneràs-Holm, Louise, FaribaBaghaei, Göran Holm, Per Olof Janson, Claes Ohlsson, Malin Lönn, and Elisabet Stener-Victorin. "Coagulation and fibrinolytic disturbances in women with polycystic ovary syndrome." *The Journal of Clinical Endocrinology & Metabolism* 96, no. 4 (2011): 1068-1076.

[89] Moreno, Pedro R., Ví´ctor H. Bernardi, Julio Lo´ pez-Cue´ llar, Alvaro M. Murcia, Igor F. Palacios, Herman K. Gold, Roxana Mehran et al. "Macrophages, smooth muscle cells, and tissue factor in unstable angina: implications for cell-mediated thrombogenicity in

acute coronary syndromes." *Circulation* 94, no. 12 (1996): 3090-3097.

[90] Deanfield, John E., Julian P. Halcox, and Ton J. Rabelink. "Endothelial function and dysfunction: testing and clinical relevance." *Circulation* 115, no. 10 (2007): 1285-1295.

[91] Mina, Ashraf, Emmanuel J. Favaloro, Soma Mohammed, and Jerry Koutts. "A laboratory evaluation into the short activated partial thromboplastin time." *Blood Coagulation andFibrinolysis* 21, no. 2 (2010): 152-157.

[92] Tripodi, Armando, VeenaChantarangkul, Ida Martinelli, Paolo Bucciarelli, and Pier MannuccioMannucci. "A shortened activated partial thromboplastin time is associated with the risk of venous thromboembolism." *Blood* 104, no. 12 (2004): 3631-3634.

[93] Lippi, Giuseppe, Massimo Franchini, Giovanni Targher, Martina Montagnana, Gian Luca Salvagno, GianCesareGuidi, and Emmanuel J. Favaloro. "Epidemiological association between fasting plasma glucose and shortened APTT." *Clinical Biochemistry* 42, no. 1-2 (2009): 118-120.

[94] Barazzoni, Rocco, MichelaZanetti, G. Davanzo, E. Kiwanuka, P. Carraro, A. Tiengo, and P. Tessari. "Increased fibrinogen production in type 2 diabetic patients without detectable vascular complications: correlation with plasma glucagon concentrations." *The Journal of Clinical Endocrinology and Metabolism* 85, no. 9 (2000): 3121-3125.

[95] Hoffbrand, A. V., P. A. H. Moss, and J. E. Pettit. *Essential haematology*, 2006. Blackwell Publishing, Malden MA, pgs 5 (2006): 249.

[96] Kelly, Christopher JG, Helen Lyall, John R. Petrie, Gwyn W. Gould, John MC Connell, Ann Rumley, Gordon DO Lowe, and NaveedSattar. "A specific elevation in tissue plasminogen activator antigen in women with polycystic ovarian syndrome." *The Journal of Clinical Endocrinology and Metabolism* 87, no. 7 (2002): 3287-3290.

[97] Lin, Sun, and Guan Yongmei. "Plasminogen activator and plasma activator inhibitor-1 in young women with polycystic ovary

syndrome." *International Journal of Gynaecology and Obstetrics* 100, no. 3 (2008): 285-286.

[98] Huang, Ying, Yong Zhao, Ling Yan, Yun-HaiChuai, Ling-Ling Liu, Yi Chen, Min Li, and Ai-Ming Wang. "Changes in coagulation and fibrinolytic indices in women with polycystic ovarian syndrome undergoing controlled ovarian hyperstimulation." *International Journal of Endocrinology* 2014 (2014).

[99] Kebapcilar, Levent, CuneytEftalTaner, AyseGulKebapcilar, and Ismail Sari. "High mean platelet volume, low-grade systemic coagulation and fibrinolytic activation are associated with androgen and insulin levels in polycystic ovary syndrome." *Archives of Gynecology and Obstetrics* 280, no. 2 (2009): 187-193.

[100] Oral, B., Mermi, B., Dilek, M., Alanoğlu, G., &Sütçü, R. (2009). Thrombin activatable fibrinolysis inhibitor and other hemostatic parameters in patients with polycystic ovary syndrome. *Gynecological Endocrinology*, 25(2), 110-116.

[101] Stegenga, Michiel E., Saskia N. Van Der Crabben, Marcel Levi, Alex F. De Vos, Michael W. Tanck, Hans P. Sauerwein, and Tom Van Der Poll. "Hyperglycemia stimulates coagulation, whereas hyperinsulinemia impairs fibrinolysis in healthy humans." *Diabetes* 55, no. 6 (2006): 1807-1812.

[102] Sobel, Burton E. "Effects of glycemic control and other determinants on vascular disease in type 2 diabetes." *The American Journal of Medicine* 113, no. 6 (2002): 12-22.

[103] Meigs, James B., Murray A. Mittleman, David M. Nathan, Geoffrey H. Tofler, Daniel E. Singer, Patricia M. Murphy-Sheehy, IzabelaLipinska, Ralph B. D'Agostino, and Peter WF Wilson. "Hyperinsulinemia, hyperglycemia, and impaired hemostasis: the Framingham Offspring Study." *JAMA* 283, no. 2 (2000): 221-228.

[104] Fauser, Bart CJM, Basil C. Tarlatzis, Robert W. Rebar, Richard S. Legro, Adam H. Balen, Roger Lobo, Enrico Carmina et al. "Consensus on women's health aspects of polycystic ovary syndrome (PCOS): the Amsterdam ESHRE/ASRM-Sponsored 3rd PCOS

Consensus Workshop Group." *Fertility and Sterility* 97, no. 1 (2012): 28-38.

[105] Wu, Fredrick CW, and Arnold von Eckardstein. "Androgens and coronary artery disease." *Endocrine Reviews* 24, no. 2 (2003): 183-217.

[106] Kebapcilar, Levent, CuneytEftalTaner, AyseGulKebapcilar, AhmetAlacacioglu, and Ismail Sari. "Comparison of four different treatment regimens on coagulation parameters, hormonal and metabolic changes in women with polycystic ovary syndrome." *Archives of Gynecology and Obstetrics* 281, no. 1 (2010): 35-42.

[107] Mak, Winifred, and AnujaDokras. "Polycystic ovarian syndrome and the risk of cardiovascular disease and thrombosis." In *Seminars in Thrombosis and Hemostasis*, vol. 35, no. 07, pp. 613-620. Thieme Medical Publishers, 2009.

[108] Coppens, Michiel, Stef P. Kaandorp, and SaskiaMiddeldorp. "Inherited thrombophilias." *Obstetrics and Gynecology Clinics* 33, no. 3 (2006): 357-374.

[109] Koster, Ted, J. P. Vandenbroucke, F. R. Rosendaal, H. De Ronde, E. Briët, and Rogier M. Bertina. "Venous thrombosis due to poor anticoagulant response to activated protein C: Leiden Thrombophilia Study." *The Lancet* 342, no. 8886-8887 (1993): 1503-1506.

[110] Kujovich, Jody Lynn. "Factor v Leiden thrombophilia." *Genetics in Medicine* 13, no. 1 (2011): 1-16.

[111] Roldan, Vanessa, Ramón Lecumberri, Juan Francisco Sánchez Muñoz-Torrero, Vicente Vicente, Eduardo Rocha, Benjamin Brenner, Manuel Monreal, and RIETE Investigators. "Thrombophilia testing in patients with venous thromboembolism. Findings from the RIETE registry." *Thrombosis Research* 124, no. 2 (2009): 174-177.

[112] DeSancho, Maria T., Tanya Dorff, and Jacob H. Rand. "Thrombophilia and the risk of thromboembolic events in women on oral contraceptives and hormone replacement therapy." *Blood Coagulation and Fibrinolysis* 21, no. 6 (2010): 534-538.

[113] Prandoni, Paolo, Anthonie WA Lensing, Alberto Cogo, Stefano Cuppini, Sabina Villalta, MariarosaCarta, Anna M. Cattelan, Paola

Polistena, Enrico Bernardi, and Martin H. Prins. "The long-term clinical course of acute deep venous thrombosis." *Annals of Internal Medicine* 125, no. 1 (1996): 1-7.

[114] Prandoni, Paolo, Anthonie WA Lensing, Alberto Cogo, Stefano Cuppini, Sabina Villalta, MariarosaCarta, Anna M. Cattelan, Paola Polistena, Enrico Bernardi, and Martin H. Prins. "The long-term clinical course of acute deep venous thrombosis." *Annals of Internal Medicine* 125, no. 1 (1996): 1-7.

[115] Rosendaal, F. R., and P. H. Reitsma. "Genetics of venous thrombosis." *Journal of Thrombosis and Haemostasis* 7 (2009): 301-304.

[116] Gohil, Reya, George Peck, and Pankaj Sharma. "The genetics of venous thromboembolism." *Thrombosis and Haemostasis* 102, no. 08 (2009): 360-370.

[117] Dahlbäck, Björn. "New molecular insights into the genetics of thrombophilia. Resistance to activated protein C caused by Arg506 to Gin mutation in factor V as a pathogenic risk factor for venous thrombosis." *Thrombosis and haemostasis* 74, no. 07 (1995): 139-148.

[118] Bare, S. N., R. Poka, I. Balogh, and E. Ajzner. "Factor V Leiden as a risk factor for miscarriage and reduced fertility." *Australian and New Zealand Journal of Obstetrics and Gynaecology* 40, no. 2 (2000): 186-190.

[119] Kazerooni, Talieh, Fariborz Ghaffarpasand, Nasrin Asadi, Zahra Dehkhoda, Maryam Dehghankhalili, and Yasaman Kazerooni. "Correlation between thrombophilia and recurrent pregnancy loss in patients with polycystic ovary syndrome: A comparative study." *Journal of the Chinese Medical Association* 76, no. 5 (2013): 282-288.

[120] Ye, Zheng, Eugene HC Liu, Julian PT Higgins, Bernard D. Keavney, Gordon DO Lowe, Rory Collins, and John Danesh. "Seven haemostatic gene polymorphisms in coronary disease: meta-analysis of 66 155 cases and 91 307 controls." *The Lancet* 367, no. 9511 (2006): 651-658.

[121] Blay, Sergio Luís, João Vicente Augusto Aguiar, and Ives Cavalcante Passos. "Polycystic ovary syndrome and mental disorders: a systematic review and exploratory meta-analysis." *Neuropsychiatric Disease and Treatment* 12 (2016): 2895.

[122] Accortt, EynavElgavish, Marlene P. Freeman, and John JB Allen. "Women and major depressive disorder: clinical perspectives on causal pathways." *Journal of Women's Health* 17, no. 10 (2008): 1583-1590.

[123] Månsson, Mattias, Jan Holte, Kerstin Landin-Wilhelmsen, Eva Dahlgren, Anette Johansson, and Mikael Landén. "Women with polycystic ovary syndrome are often depressed or anxious—a case control study." *Psychoneuroendocrinology* 33, no. 8 (2008): 1132-1138.

[124] Benson, S., P. C. Arck, S. Tan, S. Hahn, K. Mann, N. Rifaie, O. E. Janssen, M. Schedlowski, and S. Elsenbruch. "Disturbed stress responses in women with polycystic ovary syndrome." *Psychoneuroendocrinology* 34, no. 5 (2009): 727-735.

[125] Rohr, Uwe D. "The impact of testosterone imbalance on depression and women's health." *Maturitas* 41 (2002): 25-46.

[126] Miller, Christopher J., Sheri L. Johnson, and Lori Eisner. "Assessment tools for adult bipolar disorder." *Clinical Psychology: Science and Practice* 16, no. 2 (2009): 188-201.

[127] Michelmore, K. F., A. H. Balen, and D. B. Dunger. "Polycystic ovaries and eating disorders: are they related?." *Human Reproduction* 16, no. 4 (2001): 765-769.

[128] Morgan, John F., Sara E. McCluskey, Joan N. Brunton, and J. Hubert Lacey. "Polycystic ovarian morphology and bulimia nervosa: a 9-year follow-up study." *Fertility and Sterility* 77, no. 5 (2002): 928-931.

[129] Borghi, Lidia, Daniela Leone, Elena Vegni, Valentina Galiano, Corina Lepadatu, Patrizia Sulpizio, and Emanuele Garzia. "Psychological distress, anger and quality of life in polycystic ovary syndrome: associations with biochemical, phenotypicalandsociodemographic factors." *Journal of Psychosomatic Obstetrics and Gynecology* 39, no. 2 (2018): 128-137.

[130] Cooney, Laura G., and AnujaDokras. "Depression and anxiety in polycystic ovary syndrome: etiology and treatment." *Current Psychiatry Reports* 19, no. 11 (2017): 1-10.

INDEX

#

5α-dihydrotestosterone, 52, 83, 84

A

abdominal obesity, 7, 8, 47, 49
abortion, 13
acanthosis nigricans, 90, 110, 134
acid, 9, 17, 19, 35, 50, 63, 70, 101, 142
acne, viii, 38, 77, 79, 82, 83, 84, 85, 93, 107, 108, 130, 131, 149, 150
acne vulgaris, 107, 108
activated partial thromboplastin time, 145, 163
adhesion, 5, 37, 45, 49, 138, 139, 140
adipogenesis, 141
adiponectin, 8, 32, 35, 68, 70, 121, 138, 142, 143, 151, 158
adipose, 4, 8, 48, 50, 52, 100, 102, 134, 141, 156, 157
adipose tissue, 4, 8, 48, 50, 52, 100, 102, 134, 141, 157

adiposity, 8, 9, 10, 74, 89
adolescents, 19, 33, 80, 81, 84, 106, 108
adrenal gland, 82, 96, 131
adrenal hyperplasia, 80, 81
adulthood, viii, 3, 77, 84, 102
age, 3, 13, 29, 34, 36, 49, 51, 84, 91, 94, 95, 103, 129, 148, 150
alopecia, 82, 85, 86, 93, 108, 130, 131
alpha-tocopherol, 25
androgen, 3, 10, 12, 45, 50, 54, 79, 81, 82, 83, 84, 86, 95, 97, 100, 102, 114, 116, 129, 131, 132, 137, 147, 149, 152, 164
androgenic alopecia, 82, 85, 131
androgens, vii, 2, 18, 19, 37, 51, 71, 72, 82, 84, 90, 96, 99, 100, 102, 118, 131, 132, 134, 165
androstenedione, 12, 96, 97, 98, 131
aneuploidy, 61
angiogenesis, 32
angiotensin II, 46
antagonism, 159
anticoagulant, 26, 148, 165
anti-inflammatories, 14

Index

anti-inflammatory, vii, viii, 2, 12, 20, 29, 32, 33, 35, 39, 41, 66, 68, 70, 74, 75, 138, 142, 143
anti-inflammatory agents, vii, viii, 2
anti-inflammatory diet, 41, 74, 75
antioxidant, vii, viii, 2, 7, 9, 12, 13, 15, 16, 18, 20, 21, 23, 25, 26, 27, 29, 31, 33, 35, 39, 50, 55, 60, 61, 62, 63, 65, 66, 124
antioxidants, viii, 2, 6, 9, 14, 15, 20, 25, 31, 42, 46, 54, 56, 65
antral follicle, 11, 12, 97
anxiety, 14, 87, 93, 112, 130, 150, 168
anxiety disorder, 150
apoptosis, 6, 8, 12, 13, 43, 53, 55
arginine, 7, 147, 148
ascorbic acid, 26, 63
assessment, 10, 52, 69, 90, 91, 104, 114
assisted reproductive technology (ART), viii, 2, 5, 8, 13, 14, 15, 17, 18, 19, 20, 22, 23, 25, 28, 33, 38, 40, 41, 44, 55, 57, 58, 61, 64, 69
asymmetric dimethyl arginine (AMDA), 7
asymptomatic, 144
atherogenesis, 134
atherosclerosis, 92, 138, 139, 140, 141, 156, 157
atorvastatin, 37, 72
autoimmune disease, vii, 2, 3
autosomal dominant, 101

B

bacterial infection, 38
behavioral change, 40
beneficial effect, 15, 20, 25, 29, 34, 35, 38
benefits, 22, 24, 28
bilateral, 78, 105, 152
binding globulin, 40, 100, 102, 118
bioavailability, 67, 132
biochemistry, 45, 66, 70, 106
biomarker, 4, 5

biomarkers, 22, 24, 30, 60, 62, 66, 104, 119
biosynthesis, 97, 116
biosynthetic pathways, 101
bipolar disorder, 150, 167
birth rate, 18, 20, 24, 27, 28, 33, 41
birth weight, 94, 103
Bisphenol A, 102, 117, 122, 124
Bisphenol A (BPA), 117, 124
blood, vii, viii, 2, 10, 13, 15, 26, 33, 91, 104, 130, 131, 132, 133, 137, 139, 143, 144, 145, 146, 162
blood circulation, 15, 131, 137, 144, 145
blood clot, 143, 144
blood flow, 26, 130, 143
blood pressure, 131, 139
blood supply, 144
blood vessels, 143, 144, 145
body fat, 48
body image, 14, 85, 130, 150
body mass index, 4, 44, 89, 158
body weight, 17, 24, 60, 62, 89, 94, 110

C

cancer, ix, 6, 46, 47, 50, 51, 95, 104, 113, 123, 124, 128
candidates, 29, 30, 65
carbohydrate, viii, 2
carcinogenesis, 46
cardiovascular disease, 6, 14, 28, 42, 46, 87, 88, 90, 92, 104, 111, 118, 119, 120, 160, 165
cardiovascular diseases, 28, 87, 88, 90, 92, 104, 160
cardiovascular problems, vii, 2, 3
cardiovascular risk, 88, 91, 110, 122, 158
cell adhesion molecules (CAMs), 5, 45, 138, 140
cell culture, 39
cell death, 6, 29
cell differentiation, 70

Index

central nervous system, 100
cholesterol, 8, 35, 36, 39, 90, 97, 131, 135, 140, 156
chronic heart failure, 140
circulation, 32, 104, 119
cleavage, 11, 13, 60, 97, 144, 147
clinical application, 4
clinical oncology, 113
clinical presentation, ix, 78, 96, 99
clinical symptoms, x, 3, 30, 66, 82, 128, 151
clinical trials, 18, 19, 22, 30, 31
coagulation cascade, ix, 128, 134, 143, 146, 147, 149
coagulation cascade pathway, 128, 134, 143, 146, 147, 149
coenzyme, 21, 36, 61, 62
coenzyme Q10 (CoQ10), 15, 23, 61, 62
colorectal cancer, 124
combination therapy, 36
complications, vii, ix, 3, 7, 8, 14, 31, 50, 67, 78, 87, 88, 93, 102, 112, 113, 128, 148, 149, 150, 151, 154, 160, 163
congenital adrenal hyperplasia, 80, 81, 102, 117, 129
consensus, 25, 79, 105, 153
contraceptives, 69, 121, 143, 165
control group, 17, 22, 24, 25, 26, 36, 37, 38, 41
controlled trials, 31, 58, 60, 61, 71, 72
coronary angioplasty, 45
coronary artery disease, 64, 165
correlation, 29, 57, 138, 141, 145, 163
counseling, ix, 25, 128, 151
c-reactive protein (CRP), viii, 2, 4, 6, 22, 35, 39, 42, 44, 138
cross-sectional study, 32, 44, 106
culture media, 15, 21
culture medium, 29
cycles, viii, 2, 11, 13, 14, 19, 20, 22, 23, 25, 28, 34, 38, 40, 44, 57, 59, 69, 86, 99, 130
cyclophosphamide, 62
cysteine, 15, 20, 58, 59

cytochrome, 97, 100
cytokines, vii, x, 2, 6, 27, 32, 35, 43, 44, 128, 138, 139, 140, 141, 143, 151, 157, 159

D

data analysis, 17, 35, 37
d-dimer, 146, 147, 151
deep vein thrombosis, 143, 161
deep venous thrombosis, 166
defects, 9, 26, 98, 100, 133
deficiency, 64, 102, 118
degradation, 104, 145, 146, 156
demographic factors, 168
dephosphorylation, 133
depression, 14, 87, 93, 130, 150, 167
dermatology, 107, 110
developing countries, 88
diabetes, 3, 5, 6, 14, 17, 28, 31, 33, 39, 42, 45, 46, 51, 52, 60, 64, 67, 69, 70, 71, 73, 87, 89, 91, 92, 94, 95, 103, 104, 109, 110, 111, 112, 114, 115, 118, 120, 121, 123, 124, 131, 139, 154, 156, 158, 159, 160, 164
diabetic patients, 163
diagnostic criteria, 47, 78, 79, 80, 81, 105, 129, 152, 153
diet, viii, 2, 27, 40, 41, 74, 75, 101
differential diagnosis, 106
diseases, 7, 103, 121, 122, 137, 138, 139, 152
disorder, viii, ix, 9, 77, 78, 79, 81, 82, 87, 93, 104, 127, 129, 130, 137, 150, 151
dissatisfaction, 93
disseminated intravascular coagulation, 143, 161
Disseminated intravascular coagulation, 161
distribution, 48, 84, 155
DNA, 6, 21, 23, 29, 46, 60, 148
DNA damage, 6, 22

drug resistance, 125
drug therapy, 59
drug treatment, 147
drugs, 33, 69, 113, 147
dyslipidemia, vii, 2, 3, 7, 8, 9, 20, 49, 87, 89, 90, 92, 103, 110, 131, 134, 135, 136, 137
dysmenorrhea, 130

E

eating disorders, 14, 87, 93, 150, 167
embryo quality, 13, 17, 19, 21, 55, 60, 61
emotional distress, 93
emotional well-being, 130
empty follicle syndrome, 12, 13
endocrine, viii, ix, 30, 37, 43, 58, 59, 75, 77, 78, 82, 102, 104, 115, 117, 124, 128, 129, 151, 153
endocrinology, 56, 57, 60, 62, 69, 70, 71, 106, 107, 111, 114, 116, 117, 118, 119, 120, 158, 159
endocrinopathy, vii, 2, 3, 14, 43, 106
endothelial cells, 138, 160
endothelial dysfunction, 5, 45, 92, 137, 139, 140, 141
environment, 3, 25, 26, 36, 95, 102
environmental effects, 90
environmental factors, ix, 78, 82, 101, 102
enzyme, 36, 53, 61, 62, 96, 100, 122
epidemiology, 108, 114
epigenetic alterations, 6
epigenetic factors, 101, 103, 104
epithelial ovarian cancer, 95
estrogen, 26, 95, 98, 99
ethnicity, ix, 78, 81, 84, 86
etiology, viii, ix, 2, 8, 84, 101, 128, 129, 146, 168
euglycemic clamp technique, 90, 134

evidence, 14, 16, 19, 20, 22, 26, 27, 28, 29, 30, 33, 36, 40, 43, 56, 67, 69, 70, 102, 118, 119, 156
exposure, 27, 34, 102

F

factor V Leiden, 128, 147, 148, 149, 166
family history, 91, 95
family physician, 108
fasting, 10, 24, 89, 90, 92, 123, 131, 163
fasting glucose, 89, 90, 92, 131
fat, 18, 82, 91, 134, 135, 155
fatty acids, 15, 21, 35, 42, 70, 91, 133, 135, 138
fertility, 12, 15, 17, 18, 23, 25, 27, 29, 31, 33, 35, 37, 40, 42, 53, 56, 57, 61, 63, 89, 113, 161, 166
fertility rate, 36, 40
fertilization, 5, 11, 13, 17, 18, 21, 23, 25, 29, 41, 53, 55, 57, 58, 62, 64, 65, 66, 70, 95
fetal development, 102
fetal growth, 119
fibrin, 144, 145, 146
fibrinogen, 42, 144, 163
fibrinolytic, 145, 146, 162, 164
folic acid, 16, 17, 19, 65
follicle, viii, 2, 11, 12, 13, 17, 31, 54, 84, 85, 98, 115
follicular fluid, viii, 2, 5, 7, 12, 13, 17, 18, 44, 45, 47, 55, 65, 98, 104
folliculogenesis, viii, ix, 2, 3, 11, 31, 43, 53, 78, 142
formation, 11, 12, 15, 83, 84, 99, 131, 143, 144, 145, 146, 147, 148, 162
free radicals, 6, 15, 31

G

gene expression, 17, 18, 30, 39, 65, 66, 68, 103, 122
genes, 27, 36, 40, 44, 50, 101, 117, 121, 122, 136
genetic factors, 90, 101
genetic predisposition, 84
gestational age, 87, 94, 119
gestational diabetes, 17, 87, 89, 91, 102, 112, 118
glucocorticoids, 51
gluconeogenesis, 139
glucose, vii, viii, ix, 2, 3, 5, 9, 10, 17, 24, 27, 31, 32, 33, 36, 49, 52, 61, 62, 71, 73, 89, 91, 99, 100, 109, 110, 111, 128, 133, 135, 137, 139, 140, 141, 158, 159, 160, 163
glucose tolerance, 71, 89, 92, 109, 110, 111, 158
GLUT4 (glucose transporter 4), 5, 44, 68, 100, 140
glutathione, 7, 8, 9, 15, 49
glutathione peroxidase (GPx), 7, 8, 15, 49
gonadotropin-releasing hormone, 114, 119
gonadotropins, 14, 34, 37, 56, 71, 99, 142
granulosa cells (GCs), viii, 2, 11, 12, 13, 17, 18, 19, 40, 52, 53, 54, 55, 96, 97, 99, 116
growth, 10, 22, 46, 50, 51, 78, 83, 85, 100, 103, 116, 119, 130
growth factor, 10, 46, 50, 51, 100, 116
growth hormone, 51

H

hair follicle, 85
hair loss, 85, 108
harmful effects, 6, 22
health, vii, viii, x, 67, 77, 87, 88, 93, 102, 105, 111, 113, 128, 149, 153, 155, 164, 167
health care, 88
health problems, 87
health risks, vii, ix, 78, 105, 153
hepatocytes, 136, 138, 140
herbal medicine, 42
heterogeneity, vii, ix, x, 3, 14, 78, 104, 128, 130
heterozygote, 148
high blood cholesterol, 154
high density lipoprotein, 90
high-density lipoprotein cholesterol (HDL-C), 8, 9, 124
hirsutism, vii, viii, 2, 30, 32, 36, 38, 77, 78, 79, 81, 82, 83, 85, 93, 107, 129, 131, 149, 150
history, 36, 88, 107, 147
homeostasis, 10, 24, 101, 139, 144
homocysteine, 49, 92, 155
hormonal imbalance, vii, x, 2, 3, 12, 128, 135, 146, 151
hormone, 11, 18, 40, 51, 52, 53, 54, 74, 95, 96, 100, 101, 102, 115, 118, 133, 158, 165
hormone levels, 115
human, viii, 2, 18, 25, 29, 33, 49, 50, 53, 54, 55, 57, 62, 65, 69, 73, 102, 115, 116, 119, 125, 146, 158, 159, 160, 162
human chorionic gonadotropin, 119
human development, 102
human health, 29, 65
hyperandrogenism, v, vii, 1, 2, 3, 10, 15, 49, 51, 54, 71, 79, 81, 82, 83, 85, 88, 90, 92, 96, 99, 101, 102, 104, 106, 110, 114, 116, 117, 118, 119, 123, 125, 128, 129, 131, 133, 135, 136, 137, 138, 141, 146, 147, 155
hypercholesterolemia, 8
hyperglycemia, 9, 49, 51, 54, 69, 137, 146, 159, 164
hyperinsulinemia, x, 9, 10, 12, 16, 49, 88, 89, 95, 99, 103, 128, 133, 136, 139, 146, 151, 164

hyperinsulinism, 46, 119
hyperlipidemia, 48, 71
hyperplasia, 5, 12
hyperprolactinemia, 80, 81
hypertension, 14, 31, 46, 50, 87, 92, 94, 95, 103, 131, 137
hypertriglyceridemia, 90
hypertrophy, 97, 138
hypothalamus, x, 99, 128, 151
hypothesis, 13, 25, 28, 103, 110, 114, 117, 155
hypoxia-inducible factor, 6

I

idiopathic, 41, 62, 80, 81
immunopathogenesis, 3
impaired glucose tolerance (IGT), 71, 89, 91, 109, 110, 111
improvements, 16, 19, 21, 22, 24, 25, 30, 31, 33, 36, 38, 39, 40, 41, 42, 93
in vitro, 5, 22, 39, 48, 55, 58, 62, 64, 65, 66, 70, 137, 161
in vitro fertilization (IVF), 5, 11, 13, 16, 18, 19, 21, 23, 25, 26, 28, 29, 30, 34, 35, 37, 41, 45, 52, 55, 56, 57, 58, 61, 62, 63, 64, 65, 66, 69, 70, 71, 74
individuals, 5, 82, 93, 104, 138, 146, 148
induction, 3, 5, 7, 14, 16, 20, 22, 24, 27, 33, 43, 61, 69, 70
infertility, vii, viii, ix, 1, 2, 3, 8, 11, 14, 18, 20, 23, 26, 41, 43, 49, 52, 55, 59, 60, 61, 62, 66, 73, 74, 77, 82, 86, 93, 94, 95, 104, 108, 113, 114, 115, 128, 130, 148, 149, 150
inflammation, viii, ix, 2, 3, 4, 5, 6, 7, 8, 9, 10, 11, 12, 14, 22, 24, 30, 31, 32, 35, 37, 38, 42, 43, 44, 45, 46, 47, 49, 50, 51, 53, 60, 62, 66, 72, 84, 101, 128, 137, 138, 139, 140, 141, 156, 157, 158, 159, 162
inflammation markers, 128, 138

inflammatory bowel disease, 160
inflammatory cells, 142
inflammatory disease, 7, 139
inflammatory mediators, viii, 2, 4, 6, 37, 71
inflammatory responses, 4
inheritance, 86, 101, 147
inhibition, 31, 68, 103, 133
inhibitor, viii, 2, 98, 124, 146, 163, 164
injury, iv, 29, 46, 48, 139, 143, 144
inositol, 10, 15, 16, 17, 56, 57, 58, 59, 65, 69
insomnia, 18
insulin, vii, viii, ix, 2, 3, 9, 10, 12, 14, 15, 16, 17, 19, 20, 21, 22, 24, 27, 29, 31, 32, 33, 35, 36, 37, 38, 39, 44, 45, 46, 48, 49, 50, 51, 52, 53, 54, 59, 60, 64, 65, 66, 68, 72, 73, 78, 87, 88, 89, 90, 91, 92, 94, 97, 100, 101, 102, 104, 109, 110, 114, 115, 116, 117, 118, 119, 123, 124, 128, 131, 133, 134, 135, 136, 137, 138, 139, 140, 141, 142, 145, 146, 147, 154, 155, 156, 157, 158, 159, 160, 164
insulin receptor substrate (IRS), 10, 31, 100, 133, 140, 142
insulin resistance, v, vii, viii, ix, 1, 2, 3, 9, 10, 14, 15, 42, 44, 45, 46, 48, 50, 51, 52, 53, 59, 60, 66, 68, 87, 88, 89, 90, 91, 92, 94, 99, 100, 101, 102, 109, 110, 115, 116, 117, 118, 119, 120, 121, 123, 128, 131, 133, 137, 140, 146, 154, 155, 156, 157, 158, 160
insulin sensitivity, 9, 16, 33, 35, 37, 38, 46, 50, 54, 64, 68, 72, 73, 90, 138, 139, 140, 141, 145
insulin signaling, 9, 10, 50, 100, 133, 141
interleukin, viii, 2, 4, 5, 43, 44, 45, 51, 139, 143, 151, 158, 159
interleukin-1beta, 139, 158
intervention, ix, 22, 25, 27, 30, 37, 40, 41, 42, 52, 73, 74, 104, 128, 151

K

kinase activity, 140, 141

L

L-arginine, 15
L-carnitine, 21, 22, 60
lifestyle, vii, viii, ix, 2, 3, 33, 35, 40, 41, 43, 73, 74, 75, 78, 92, 93, 101, 106, 128, 151
lifestyle modification, vii, viii, 2, 33, 35, 40, 41, 73, 75, 92
ligand, 136, 138, 142
lipid metabolism, ix, 65, 128, 131, 135, 136, 139, 159
lipid peroxidation, 23, 31
lipogenesis, 133
lipolysis, 91, 133, 134, 135
liver, 14, 39, 50, 100, 104, 133, 136, 138, 140, 144
low-density lipoprotein cholesterol (LDL-C), 8, 35, 124
low-grade inflammation, v, vii, 1, 2, 5, 8, 157
luteinizing hormone, 10, 51, 52, 54, 96, 115, 116, 119
lymphocytes, 30, 140
lymphoma, 159

M

macrophages, 138, 139, 140, 142, 144, 156
malondialdehyde (MDA), 7, 8, 9, 10, 12, 13, 22, 124
mammalian cells, 6
management, viii, ix, 3, 6, 14, 41, 67, 69, 78, 93, 95, 107, 108, 109, 128, 130, 151
measurement, 37, 38, 134, 145, 162
medical, 75, 93, 128, 147
medical science, 75
medicine, 14, 41, 63, 109, 111, 113, 154, 159
melatonin, 15, 16, 18, 19, 57, 58, 65
mellitus, 17, 33, 39, 42, 87, 91, 104, 111, 112, 118, 131, 154, 160
menstrual cycles, 16, 40, 86, 89
menstruation, 20, 25
mental disorder, 167
mental health, 60, 66, 104, 111
messenger ribonucleic acid, 53
messenger RNA, 103
meta-analysis, 4, 20, 22, 23, 28, 34, 35, 37, 39, 40, 44, 47, 49, 58, 59, 60, 61, 62, 64, 70, 71, 72, 73, 91, 92, 93, 94, 106, 109, 112, 113, 116, 148, 166, 167
metabolic change, 165
metabolic disorder, 7, 14, 43, 89, 140, 155, 156, 157
metabolic disturbances, 52
metabolic dysfunction, ix, 42, 102, 128
metabolic pathways, 100
metabolic syndrome, ix, 8, 28, 42, 48, 49, 88, 103, 104, 109, 121, 123, 124, 128, 131, 151, 157, 158, 160
metabolism, 6, 9, 24, 27, 29, 31, 33, 35, 36, 52, 56, 57, 61, 62, 63, 73, 82, 91, 99, 100, 103, 106, 111, 117, 118, 119, 133, 159
metformin, 16, 20, 21, 24, 25, 30, 32, 33, 35, 36, 37, 38, 40, 42, 43, 58, 59, 60, 68, 69, 70, 71, 72, 73, 75
micronutrients, 30
miscarriage, 11, 16, 24, 28, 34, 36, 89, 94, 166
mitochondrial dysfunction, 7, 8, 30, 100
molecules, 5, 26, 45, 49, 137, 138, 140, 160
mononuclear cells, vii, 2, 49, 51, 137, 140
morphology, 31, 52, 79, 81, 87, 108, 129, 167
mortality, 87, 88, 91, 161
mutation, 118, 147, 148, 149, 166
myocardial infarctions, 148

myo-inositol (MYO), 15, 16, 17, 19, 56, 57, 58, 65

N

N-acetyl cysteine (NAC), 9, 20, 58, 59
neurodegenerative diseases, 122
nuclear factor-κB (NFκB), viii, 2
nutrition, 42, 63, 70, 74, 75, 101, 103

O

obesity, vii, viii, 2, 3, 4, 5, 6, 7, 8, 9, 10, 14, 19, 40, 42, 45, 46, 47, 48, 49, 50, 64, 75, 83, 86, 87, 88, 89, 91, 92, 93, 94, 95, 101, 103, 109, 110, 113, 114, 117, 119, 124, 130, 131, 135, 137, 138, 140, 144, 150, 154, 157, 158, 160
obsessive-compulsive disorder, 150
oligomenorrhea, viii, 77, 86, 88
oligoovulation, 3
omega-3, 15, 35, 42, 70
omega-3-polyunsaturzted fatty acids, 15, 35
oocyte, viii, 2, 8, 11, 12, 13, 16, 17, 18, 19, 21, 22, 25, 32, 36, 52, 53, 57, 58, 60, 61, 139, 158
oocyte maturity, 13
oocyte quality, viii, 2, 8, 12, 17, 18, 32, 52, 57, 58
osteoprotegerin, 6, 45
ovarian cancer, 7, 95, 113
ovarian dysfunction, 11, 13, 18, 38, 50, 51, 53, 79, 86, 99, 114, 118, 157
ovarian tumor, 95, 113
ovaries, 3, 10, 11, 12, 25, 27, 32, 48, 52, 53, 54, 78, 79, 80, 82, 90, 96, 100, 104, 105, 114, 115, 116, 117, 128, 131, 133, 137, 141, 152, 167
overweight, 4, 40, 41, 48, 49, 68, 74, 75, 88, 94, 109, 113, 160

ovulation, 3, 5, 11, 16, 20, 22, 24, 25, 27, 33, 38, 40, 60, 61, 69, 70, 72, 86, 89, 99, 100, 139, 142, 159
oxidation, 8, 21, 23, 31, 138
oxidative damage, 15
oxidative stress (OS), v, viii, 1, 2, 6, 7, 8, 9, 10, 12, 13, 14, 20, 22, 24, 27, 30, 43, 45, 46, 47, 48, 49, 50, 51, 52, 54, 55, 58, 60, 62, 63, 65, 66, 70, 122, 137, 157
oxygen, 21, 51

P

paraoxonase-1 (PON1), 7, 122, 124
pathogenesis, v, vii, ix, x, 1, 2, 5, 9, 10, 11, 12, 14, 43, 78, 84, 96, 97, 99, 102, 103, 107, 109, 110, 114, 117, 128, 133, 137, 141, 151, 155, 161
pathogens, 125
pathophysiological, viii, 2, 58, 96, 99, 104, 108, 145
pathophysiological roles, viii, 2
pathophysiology, viii, 2, 8, 53, 57, 82, 107, 140, 157
peroxisome proliferator-activated receptor gamma, 141
pharmacological treatment, 92
pharmacology, 59, 66, 67
phenotype, 7, 88, 94, 101, 104, 113, 114, 152
phenotypes, ix, 9, 28, 30, 78, 79, 89, 92, 94, 102
phosphorylation, 31, 67, 100, 117, 133, 138, 140, 142, 154
placebo, 15, 16, 20, 21, 23, 25, 26, 27, 29, 30, 32, 33, 34, 35, 37, 38, 39, 60, 62, 63, 68, 70, 71, 72, 73
platelet aggregation, 6, 31, 67
polycystic ovarian morphology (PCOM), 80, 81, 87, 108, 129, 167
polymenorrhoea, 86

polymorphism, 82, 121, 122, 124
polyunsaturated fat, 141
polyunsaturated fatty acids, 141
population, 34, 41, 81, 88, 91, 92, 113, 124, 142, 144, 147, 150, 152, 161
pregnancy, viii, ix, 2, 5, 13, 14, 16, 18, 20, 21, 23, 25, 26, 27, 28, 33, 34, 40, 42, 55, 60, 65, 69, 74, 86, 87, 89, 93, 102, 112, 118, 122, 128, 148, 166
pregnancy complications, ix, 87, 93, 94, 102, 112, 113, 128
pregnancy loss, 13, 148, 166
prevalence, viii, x, 47, 78, 79, 80, 83, 84, 85, 88, 91, 94, 101, 102, 105, 106, 107, 109, 110, 112, 113, 117, 119, 128, 129, 130, 131, 150, 152
primary follicles, 12
progesterone, 5, 12, 27, 32, 38, 63, 79, 86, 99
prognosis, 55, 61, 119
programming, 101, 103, 118, 119
pro-inflammatory, 6, 32, 137, 138, 139, 140, 141, 143
proinflammatory cytokines, vii, 2, 27, 35
proliferation, 12, 31, 39, 43, 51, 84, 97, 157
prothrombin time, 145
psychiatric disorder, 93, 130, 149, 151
psychological distress, 150, 153
psychological implications, 93
psychological problems, 42
psychological well-being, 93, 104
psychopathology, 130
pulmonary embolism, ix, 128, 143, 161

Q

quality of life, viii, 14, 78, 79, 83, 85, 93, 104, 130, 150, 168
quercetin, 31, 66, 67, 68

R

randomized clinical trial, 16, 57, 60
reactive oxygen species (ROS), viii, 2, 3, 6, 9, 10, 12, 13, 14, 17, 25, 29, 51, 53, 54, 62, 137, 141, 159
reproduction, 7, 29, 54, 60, 62, 64, 65, 69, 74, 108, 109, 112, 113, 116, 118, 119, 139, 158
reproductive age, 78, 80, 81, 82, 87, 104, 106
researchers, 30, 31
resistance, vii, x, 2, 14, 51, 89, 91, 99, 102, 103, 109, 110, 116, 118, 121, 128, 131, 133, 137, 148, 158
resistin, 68, 121, 140, 141, 143, 151, 160, 161
response, 5, 6, 11, 24, 32, 38, 61, 89, 96, 99, 116, 131, 133, 141, 143, 144, 165
resveratrol, 38, 39, 43, 73
risk, ix, 7, 28, 34, 39, 47, 70, 78, 87, 88, 90, 91, 92, 93, 95, 104, 111, 112, 118, 123, 124, 128, 131, 135, 138, 139, 140, 141, 145, 147, 148, 149, 150, 154, 161, 163, 165, 166
risk factors, ix, 70, 78, 88, 92, 94, 95, 128, 131, 135, 140, 141, 149
ROS hypoxia-inducible factor-1 (HIF-1), 6
Rotterdam criteria, 43, 79, 80, 87, 129, 152

S

seborrhea, 82, 83, 84
sebum, 83, 84
secrete, 11, 131
secretion, ix, 12, 31, 78, 89, 95, 96, 99, 101, 132, 139, 146
selenium (Se), 29
self-esteem, 85, 87, 93, 150
sensitivity, viii, 2, 35, 99, 100, 141
serine, 100, 117, 154, 155

serum, viii, 2, 4, 5, 10, 13, 17, 24, 27, 28, 32, 35, 36, 37, 38, 39, 40, 44, 45, 62, 63, 65, 70, 74, 82, 86, 100, 118
signal transduction, 31, 116, 154
signaling pathway, 6, 7, 141
signs, viii, 13, 77, 81, 86, 130
simvastatin, 36, 38, 71, 72, 73
skeletal muscle, 70, 100, 115, 138, 154
skin, 17, 27, 82, 83, 90, 100, 107
sleep disturbance, 58
sleeping problems, 58
smooth muscle, 31, 162
social phobia, 150
socioeconomic status, 101
sodium, 29, 30, 65, 139
species, viii, 2, 6, 51, 53, 54, 62, 102
sperm, 25, 43, 47, 60
spontaneous pregnancy, 18
statins, 36, 37, 38, 72
steroidogenesis, ix, 32, 33, 52, 69, 78, 97, 98, 99, 100, 128, 132, 139, 142, 154
stimulation, 5, 13, 18, 19, 39, 43, 46, 47, 56, 58, 63, 91, 99, 100, 113, 119, 131, 132, 133, 137, 161
stress, 6, 8, 15, 39, 43, 46, 47, 50, 52, 55, 58, 63, 73, 122, 137, 149, 157, 167
strokes, 148
subfertility, 11, 56, 69
superoxide dismutase (SOD), 7, 8, 10, 15, 22, 124
supplementation, vii, viii, 2, 17, 19, 21, 23, 25, 26, 27, 28, 29, 30, 32, 35, 39, 58, 60, 61, 62, 63, 64, 65, 66, 68, 70
symptoms, vii, viii, ix, 2, 78, 86, 93, 112, 128, 130, 151
syndrome, vii, ix, 2, 3, 12, 13, 33, 43, 44, 45, 46, 47, 48, 49, 50, 51, 52, 53, 54, 55, 56, 57, 59, 60, 61, 62, 63, 64, 65, 66, 67, 68, 69, 70, 71, 72, 73, 74, 75, 78, 80, 81, 88, 90, 94, 101, 105, 106, 107, 108, 109, 110, 111, 112, 113, 114, 115, 116, 117, 118, 119, 121, 123, 124, 125, 128, 131, 137, 147, 149, 150, 152, 153, 154, 155, 157, 158, 161, 162, 164, 165, 166, 167, 168
synthesis, 15, 27, 29, 39, 65, 97, 116, 131, 133, 134, 146

T

testosterone, 4, 12, 16, 24, 27, 30, 32, 36, 37, 38, 39, 57, 62, 79, 82, 83, 84, 96, 103, 114, 116, 124, 134, 136, 145, 147, 150, 156, 167
theca cells, 10, 12, 96, 97, 99, 100, 114, 131, 133, 137, 142, 161
therapeutic effect, 31, 37, 72
therapeutic targets, 104
therapy, 15, 17, 20, 23, 26, 27, 31, 33, 35, 37, 39, 57, 59, 62, 65, 72, 159, 165
thrombophilia, 147, 148, 165, 166
thrombosis, 140, 141, 143, 145, 146, 147, 148, 156, 161, 162, 165, 166
thrombus, 146, 162
thyroid, 29, 80, 81
tissue, 89, 104, 139, 144, 157, 159, 160, 162, 163
tissue factor, 144, 147, 151, 162
tissue plasminogen activator, 145, 163
TNF-α, 5, 10, 12, 22, 30, 70, 121, 122, 137, 139, 140, 141, 142
transforming growth factor, 138
treatment, vii, viii, 2, 6, 13, 14, 15, 16, 17, 18, 19, 20, 21, 22, 23, 25, 26, 28, 30, 31, 32, 33, 34, 35, 36, 38, 39, 41, 44, 52, 54, 55, 56, 57, 58, 59, 61, 62, 64, 65, 68, 70, 71, 72, 73, 77, 95, 107, 122, 130, 142, 147, 151, 152, 154, 155, 165, 168
trial, 16, 24, 27, 37, 38, 41, 57, 58, 60, 61, 62, 63, 64, 68, 70, 71, 72, 73, 74, 75
triglycerides, 8, 9, 91, 131
tumor, viii, 2, 4, 43, 44, 51, 80, 81, 102, 159

Index

tumor necrosis factor-α (TNFα), viii, 2, 22, 43, 157
type 2 diabetes, 3, 28, 64, 73, 87, 89, 91, 103, 109, 110, 111, 139, 158, 159, 160, 164
tyrosine, 31, 100, 116

U

ultrasound, 3, 79, 115
ultrastructure, 43
ultraviolet irradiation, 27
underlying mechanisms, 19, 67
unstable angina, 45, 162

V

vascular cell adhesion molecule, 5
vascular diseases, 139, 148
vascular endothelial growth factor (VEGF), 19

venous thromboembolism, 143, 163, 165, 166
visfatin, 121, 140, 143, 151, 159, 160
vitamin C, 26, 27
vitamin D, 15, 24, 25, 27, 28, 63, 64, 65
vitamin D deficiency, 28
vitamin D3, 25, 27, 28
vitamin E, 9, 24, 25, 26, 35, 62, 63
vitamins, 15, 25, 26, 27

W

weight control, 33
weight gain, 82, 88
worldwide, viii, 77, 80, 130

Z

zona pellucida, 12, 53